ROOT CAUSE MEDICINE

FOR PEOPLE WHO DON'T GET BETTER

Suffering with Cancer, Dementia, Hormonal Aging,
Inflammatory Disorders, and Obesity

GEORGE F. MORICZ, M.D.

ISBN: 979-8-218-50346-8

DISCLAIMER

The information contained in this book is intended to provide helpful and informative material on the subject addressed. It is not intended to serve as a replacement for professional medical advice. Any use of the information in this book is at the reader's discretion. The author and publisher disclaim any and all liability arising directly and indirectly from the use or application of any information contained in this book.

Table of Contents

Introduction

Why people do not get better – the question that has been on so many people's minds but never entirely comfortable asking it.

Before we can truly ask why people do not get better, we need to explore why people decline, biologically age, get sick and show up to the doctor's office saying - why can't I get better.

Who is this for?

People drained of energy and brain fog to dementia and cancer, this book will explore the latest approaches very few have heard of and even fewer have taken advantage of, but every one of you could.

In this journey, we will explore why youth is perfect health, and why antiaging regenerative medicine which is the reason you had youth in the first place. Imagine rewinding you back to youth - 20 years of age – when you had the most perfect pattern of youthful chemicals running through your brain and body. At 20 years of age, this perfect pattern of youthful chemicals was not only what you had in youth but actually gave you youth. It did not matter if you slept right, ate right, you woke up the next day and you were a sexual dynamo. Then 10, 20, 30 years later from age 20, you notice changes in your sleep, mood, energy, face and body composition. Subsequently, you dedicate a number of years troubleshooting and trying to recover what was most perfect in your youth.

Assuming that you did not develop any of the 2 biggest killers in the United States including heart disease and cancer until much later in life, the quality of your productivity, energy and enjoyable evenings is nothing like what you experienced years ago. So, what do you do?

You go to traditional doctors, complementary doctors, seek alternative approaches and research Google endlessly and try things online. If your problem is simple, maybe you get lucky, and it is not such a big problem at all. For many others the problems are more complex than a simple Band-Aid solution. And still, you may see 5 - 10 different practitioners before coming to see someone like me.

Traditional doctor approaches are failing you. Big Pharma and insurance companies act like a tow truck for your brain and body – when your car breaks down you need to get towed to the repair shop. Traditional medicine waits for you to qualify for certain diagnostic markers just like a dashboard warning light in your vehicle. Waiting for the check engine light usually means the process has been going on for a while and now we are going to offer a one-step solution. Disappointing to many and rarely successful in the long run, smart and savvy people start seeking out why they don't get better.

From the realm of metabolism, nutrition, detoxification, dementia and cancer, this book will explore the latest approaches very few have heard of and even fewer have taken advantage of, but every one of you could.

FREE GIFTS TO HELP YOU!

For those of you who enjoy video learning and discovery of Dr. Moricz' treasure trove of anti-aging secrets, please go to www.bodyhormone.com

For those of you who enjoy radio podcasts on topics you are not likely to stumble upon yourself, please visit www.georgemoricz.com

For those of you interested in discovering what are hormones, anyway, please go to www.beautychanneldoc.com

For those of you wanting to discover why most weight loss programs don't work, please visit www.gobodyhormone.com

For any comments, questions or requests for the following publications, please email us at info@bodyhormonebalance.com

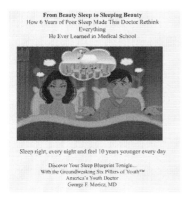

From Beauty Sleep to Sleeping Beauty
How 6 Years of Poor Sleep Made This Doctor Rethink Everything
He Ever Learned in Medical School

Sleep right, every night and feel 10 years younger every day

Discover Your Sleep Blueprint Tonight...
With the Groundbreaking Six Pillars of Youth™
America's Youth Doctor
George F. Moricz, MD

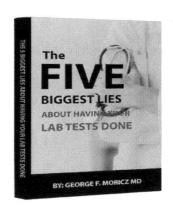

The 5 Biggest Lies about Lab Testing that are Keeping You Fat, Fatigued and Feeling "Older Than Your Years"

Investigative Report by Dr George Moricz
Doctormoricz.com

Chapter 1

Designing Success

I feel compelled to share a story that caught me 'off guard' and gave me a perspective that helped me understand something more valuable than what I thought I was really doing.

A pretty sharp lady made a confession to me—so here it goes....

Before she made the decision to come to me on the quest to get back her life, she felt like she was going to amateurs — she had every imaginable health care advisor, expert and doctor OFFER her BIG short term promises that would fix everything ... what she painfully realized (after losing lots of time, money and quality years) is that she was in the little leagues by going to technicians and mechanics WHEN instead she should have started with me "because you are reengineering my body and mind NOT just changing or throwing parts at me *like a car.* Because of this approach, I witnessed my productivity, and relationships transform themselves literally overnight which is what I was really looking for in the first place..."

Shared by one of my VIP clients, she nailed down a principle that has become more strikingly clear to other clients as well...

YOUR BODY AND MIND WERE ENGINEERED FOR YOUTH

Why am I sharing this and why now?

In a moment, I will share a story of what made me do what I do today. For many years, I had many people come to me looking for their youthful blueprint. Twenty years as a doctor I *finally* 'cracked the code' on youth with three seldom shared but very potent secrets:

ACCEPTED FACT #1: Youth is perfect health. In other words, when you had youth, it didn't matter if you slept right, ate right, you woke up the next day, you had lots of energy and you certainly didn't have sexual trouble.

ACCEPTED FACT #2: When you had youth, you had the perfect combination of natural chemicals and hormones running through your brain and body.

ACCEPTED FACT #3: When I rewind you back to your youthful blueprint, you start enjoying all the things you ONCE enjoyed about being young again.

When you had youth, you not only *had* the perfect combination of natural chemicals and hormones, but it is this very perfect combination of these natural hormones and chemicals that *gave you youth – which* is your youthful blueprint – the SECRET basis of every transformation enjoyed by my clients.

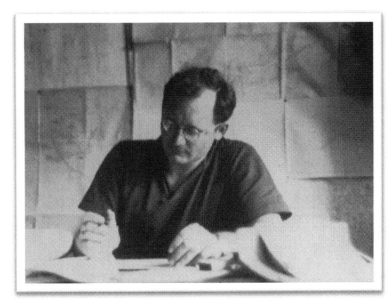

A PHOTO OF MY FATHER DESIGNING SUPERHIGHWAYS

So, what was the <u>real influence</u> as to why a doctor surgeon who was trained in traditional principles *risked everything and would* exit the comfort and convenience of a well-established medical practice, to design a superior approach for re-engineering (designing YOU back) what was perhaps the most perfect thing about you – your youthful blueprint?

It was my father.

My father was a structural engineer who dedicated himself to designing superhighways for much of his career. I grew up influenced by engineering principles, which ONLY many years later critically became a 'game changing breakthrough' for my work in helping people as a doctor. But most critical of all, what I discovered was that there was a huge advantage to having grown up as the son of an engineer with exposure to the design of highways, bridges and very impressive structures.

More specifically, the concept of designing ***blueprints*** would later be the very breakthrough and perhaps the greatest medical breakthrough that I had witnessed as a doctor. You see, if my father had been a medical doctor, I would probably have stayed within the box of usual conventional approaches. But the very day that I asked myself *"Why is it that doctors are constantly treating people with the assumption that they should be sick and come to the doctor sick and will ultimately stay sick and BELIEVE that they were never really youthfully healthy in the first place...?"*

In fact, they did have a time in their life when they had perfect health and that's what we call youth. Then I started to wonder, "What if I could take people back to this perfect combination of youthful chemicals and hormones and give them back all the things they enjoyed about being young again ...?"

Well, over time all these questions volcanically collided together and created a lot of controversy with what doctors and everyday people are taught. The one thing that was hard to argue with were RESULTS of enjoying your youthful blueprint — the life changing results that people enjoyed in their relationships, energy and ability to enjoy life the way they did years ago but now at a point in their life with acquired experience that time has given them as well.

So, it was my father's influence that made me think of **designing blueprints**. In my teenage years, I worked doing engineering drafting and *blueprints* for my father and *only many years later* did I fully appreciate how there was an *undiscovered blueprint* that everybody was walking around with but very few people were enjoying (until now of course).

That's why I believe discovering your unique custom blueprint is perhaps one of the greatest discoveries of medical science, and I am glad to have created this system to share for 'smart and savvy people' who come to me from all over the country.

In a recently released book *Applied Minds: How Engineers Think* by Guru Madhaven, the author says that engineers have been recognized as heroes in designing everything like our: iPhone, microprocessors, computer codes, pharmaceuticals, rockets, electrical systems and air traffic control. More specifically, the "golden basis" to all these engineering marvels is three separate but equally unifying principles:

First: Good engineers create *structures* so they can understand, preemptively, the context and value of any given problem and solution.

Second: After that, they acknowledge *constraints* whether of money or politics or available materials, that they must work within or somehow supersede.

Third: They deftly evaluate *trade-offs* so that they can formulate the most effective application for a given situation.

So, you may already be wondering WHY is it that so many people who are *fortunate to discover their very own youthful blueprint* 10, 20, 30 years since they were actually youthful YET "still stay stuck" UNNECESSARILY even though they do not have to?

The ANSWER for this is the very reason that they could not transform their productivity, relationships and lead a very BIG LIFE in the first place:

THEY ARE STUCK IN NON-ENGINEERING PRINCIPLES

In the left-handed box **(figure 1)** below, they have been told so many times over and over again and have erroneously convinced themselves that they should start searching for a solution of constraints evaluating trade-offs, limitations and self-doubt to seal and almost guarantee failure.

The success of using sound engineering principles can be summarized in a 3-step model as noted in **figure 2**. The first principle of designing an engineering structure comprehensively matches the underlying problem with a solution. It is the first and only step taken first. It is only after this first step is developed that the second principle of constraints, be it money, preference or truly defined limitations are applied to the first principle of a structured problem-solution. Then, the third engineering principle of evaluating trade-offs so that the most effective application can be formulated for a given situation.

Most people arrive to me "**STUCK**" in the left-handed column approach:

Figure 1 – One Step model.

In most cases, they have never been shown the successful 3-step engineering model of designing a success blueprint. So, they are continuously and religiously "**STUCK**" in a One-Step non-engineered approach that has already compromised their chances of success for a very BIG LIFE.

THE INSURANCE BAND-AID APPROACH

(1-Step Non-Engineering Model)

DESIGNING SUCCESS BLUEPRINT

(3-Step Engineering Model)

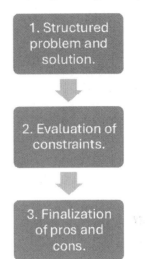

1. Start and finish with solution by constraints.

(Figure 1)
Aging before your time

(Figure 2)
Look, feel, and perform like you did in your twenties

So, how can you "IMMEDIATELY benefit from the secret" that took me twenty years to discover as a doctor and a lifetime of learning from my father so that you, too, can now lead a very BIG LIFE with supercharged relationships and productivity RIGHT NOW.

Discovering the above 3-step principles for designing success is perhaps your key to unlocking everything that I have helped you discover with your youthful blueprint. In other words, the most fortunate of people even when given their youthful blueprint (who are "stuck" in a non-engineered one step principle) shown in **figure** 1 will never fully enjoy the benefits of their youthful blueprint.

On the other hand, with a healthy sense of skepticism by opening your mind to a 3-step engineering design for success **(figure 2)** applied to your individualized youthful blueprint practically guarantees your odds for success.

Let me warn you - time and time again there are those who are given their blueprint, who stare at their blueprint, who acknowledge that it exists, who wish to think differently about their blueprint, and delay the inevitable only to eventually realize that *"facts are stubborn things"* – the quicker, the sooner that you take action on rediscovering your youthful blueprint saves years of frustration and puts you light years ahead for taking years off your age even when nothing else has never worked. Now, you have the golden key for how I can re-engineer success with your youthful blueprint so you can now enjoy all the things that you once enjoyed about being young again. There is only power in action so stop delaying any further.

Look, feel, and perform like you did in your 20's in record time even when nothing has ever worked.

Chapter 2

Youth is Perfect Health

Let's take a moment to look back at when you were twenty years of age. That's right. Rewind back to your 20-year-old image of yourself. Remember how you felt? Remember how you looked? Remember the energy you had and how you looked forward to every day? When you were 20 years old, you didn't have to eat right, and you didn't have to sleep right. You woke up feeling great nearly every day, and you certainly didn't have any sexual trouble.

This is the basis for the **Root Cause Based Medicine** and my custom designed **Youthful Blueprint System™**. In other words, you have a 20-year-old blueprint. And with this blueprint that you had at 20, you had possibly the best profile of hormonal balance and nutrition than you would ever have in your life. Had I met you when you were 20, I would have analyzed your weight and body composition; I would have analyzed your hormonal levels; I would have analyzed your intracellular nutrition and performed a functional assessment of your health. Then, later in life, when you decided that things weren't going so well, another assessment would be performed, measuring, once again, weight and body composition and hormonal and nutritional profiles, along with a functional assessment of your health.

Then, comparisons would be made, and re-adjustments would be recommended.

Imagine if you will that an architect has the blueprints for a building. Then over time, with shifts in land, as well as settling of the house and the wear and tear on the structure of the building, a reassessment would have to be made to return things to the original blueprint. Well, this is no different than returning you to your 20-year-old blueprint.

When clients come to me in their late 20's and early 30's, they may be experiencing a nosedive in their hormones. Half the people I see with no symptoms at all actually demonstrate changes at the level of the ***cell and blood hormones***, which are already starting the eventual nosedive of perfect hormonal balance and nutritional protection they once enjoyed.

However, what is more common in conventional medicine is to wait until men and women are well into their 40's and 50's and beyond before intervening.

People are all too familiar with the terms **MENOPAUSE** and **ANDROPAUSE**. This chapter will not spend time arguing the exact definitions and whether there is complete hormonal cessation in men and women. But what is important is the timing of the intervention. In other words, what is the benefit of waiting until there is a complete nosedive in hormones and nutrition when someone has chronologically aged, rather than attacking the issue well before health problems arrive?

What is all this talk about *hormones*, what are we really trying to measure? When speaking about hormones, important categories include:

- Reproductive hormones

- Stress gland hormones

- Thyroid hormones

- Pancreatic hormones

Other non-hormonal measurements, which are interrelated, include **body composition**, which specifically looks at the amount of muscle and fat in the body.

It is well known that when people are aging before their years, they not only have changes in cognitive function, a decrease in energy, an increase in fatigue, but also an increase in weight, and, in particular, a decrease in muscle and an increase in fat.

In twenty years, the standard of care is likely to involve an analysis of body composition, where the fifth vital sign will include measurement of body fat percentage. In other words, people will not only know their blood pressure, pulse, temperature and weight, but they will also know their body fat percentage. **A lot could be said about this, but for practical purposes, knowing body fat percentage is already signifying the early signs of inflammation in the body and hormonal imbalance**.

So, what are people doing to address this, and what is the medical profession recommending?

Well, we all know that people will use caffeine, stimulants and any over-the-counter fix, including the use of sugar, to help them fix issues with energy, focus and metabolism. When the individual actually seeks medical help, it is not uncommon to be placed on stimulants for focus and weight control. It is not uncommon to be prescribed antidepressants and sedatives to help mood and coping issues with daily life, and it is not uncommon to be prescribed sleep aids to help with disruptive sleep.

By the time somebody reaches age 50, the medical establishment is well-versed in the use of synthetic hormones for diagnoses such as **MENOPAUSE** and **ANDROPAUSE**. It is beyond the scope of this book to cover the pros and cons of these approaches but mentioning them brings attention to the fact that "this" is the usual chronology.

I would suggest that, whether it is over the counter or prescribed, that intervention should start between the ages of 30 and 50 when strides can be made, and not in the 50+ age category after a lot of ground has already been lost.

Let's talk about some of the mechanisms of aging.

Everywhere you turn, you hear about "healthy aging," or "anti-aging." Just for a point of reference, there are a number of different mechanisms that have been proposed to stop the aging process, including reversing damage from free radicals, inflammation, insulin resistance and mitochondrial dysfunction. Put simply, there are molecules called free radicals that require neutralization, so they don't cause damage. There are chemicals related to inflammation that are spewed from everything from fat cells all the way to the breakdown of certain ingested foods. Still further, there is the issue of pre-diabetes, which eventually can manifest itself as full diabetes. And finally, there are energy powerhouses within the cells called mitochondria, which, as they become less efficient, are associated with loss of energy.

What we are discussing here could be summed up as the diagnosis for aging.

In addition, many times, people are told that, because they are aging, there is a corresponding drop in their hormones. It is not to suggest that the nosedive in hormones described earlier is responsible for every seen and unseen hidden ill of aging. But what if the hormonal nosedive were responsible at some level for the aging process, as well?

Let me suggest it another way: Consider, if you would, that many medical problems that people are experiencing may not really be true medical problems at all! They may be a function of hormonal imbalance.

The number and different types of hormones may not be particularly important to list, identify, and write about in this short book. However, consider that, whenever hormones are not in the perfect blueprint ratio that was present in your 20's, your body may be in hormonal imbalance. Once again, as you age, there is an association with decreased hormones. So, what if the decrease in hormones is the cause of aging and all its unpleasant side effects inside and outside of your body?

A WORD OR TWO ABOUT HORMONES.

Hormones as chemical messengers serve many critical functions. The body is often considered a balance of the breakdown and buildup of tissues for proper functioning. Words such as "*anabolic*" versus "*catabolic*" are often used. Think of anabolic as rebuilding and protecting your body and catabolic as breaking down tissues, especially during signs of inflammation. So, in essence, what if hormones could regulate inflammation? There is a field called immunomodulation which essentially focuses on hormones, particularly the male-derived ones that are involved with regulation of inflammation. This actually makes a lot of sense, because you notice that as you get older you are often plagued with immune and inflammatory problems, which you were able to handle much easier earlier in life.

www.YourbeautyDoc.com

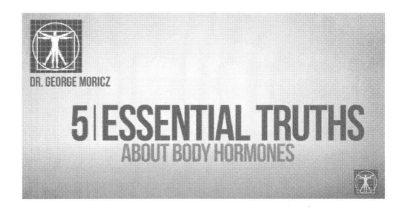

A WORD OR TWO ABOUT NUTRITION.

Earlier, these chemicals, called free radicals, were mentioned. They are responsible for cell damage and are probably heightened during exercise and while eating. Nutritional supplementation and properly balanced antioxidants with foods are thought to be protective. Nutrition is also important when looking at energy. Earlier, I mentioned *mitochondria*, which are the powerhouses within cells. It is now thought that in muscles, and to a degree in the brain, that these powerhouses may be the connection not only for energy, but the protection of the cell's longevity. So, it makes sense to see nutrition from a cell protective perspective, as well as an energy perspective, as well.

No discussion would be complete without a brief word on environmental exposures...

Everywhere you turn, you will see information on everything from toxic metals, and chemicals in the environment. It is thought that, both at the level of damaging cells, as well as disrupting hormonal balance in the body, that environmental exposure is responsible for everything from infertility, some cancers and shortened lifespan.

A holistic approach would argue that many people do not recover from traditional medical approaches because removal of these toxic exposures has not been complete. While I cannot exclude the possibility of this, it arguably makes sense to optimize hormonal balance to assist the body in helping it repair itself and improve its immune function. Certainly, as the body ages, it has to deal further with cell damage and repair.

Another perspective on aging is that it is the breaking down of most processes into inflammation and energy issues. Think about inflammation as removing offending agents in the body so that rebuilding of the tissues can occur. This can explain in simple terms everything from allergies to autoimmune diseases (i.e., rheumatoid and lupus).

With respect to energy, the brain and the body depend on proper powerhouse function so that there can be an efficient processing of nutrition to make a currency we now know as ATP. Based on breakdown of the particular processes that are involved in the transfer of nutrients and co-factors, it is evident that nutrition is critical for energy production within the cell.

So, what does anti-aging have to do with all this? Nutrition and hormonal balance are the most effective ways to attack inflammation and energy issues.

On the surface, one could evaluate body composition, skin and hair quality, and sexual function. On a deeper level, hormones and nutrition affect the immune system. An entire field of *immunomodulation* has been built on the role of hormones regulating the immune system.

Nutrition is equally important, especially when it comes to looking at foods and seeing how they affect anti-inflammatory pathways in the body. In summary, the **Root Cause Based Medicine using the Youthful Blueprint System**™ is based on complete balance of all your hormones.

Hormones can work with or against each other, which is why hormonal expertise in balancing these hormones as correlated with symptoms is performed on an individual basis. Put another way, you have a 20-year-old blueprint for both nutrition and hormones.

When it comes to handling illnesses involving issues with energy and inflammation, it is critical in the experience of this system to return an individual to the 20-year-old blueprint so that the body can best handle the processes that are causing the problem.

As an example, in conventional medicine, when people come in with issues of energy, a common culprit is the use of statin medications, which are used to attack cholesterol abnormalities. As another example, the medications used for chemotherapy and rheumatoid arthritis are often so toxic to regular cells, that they can over-suppress the immune system and make one susceptible to basic infections. Still others receive medications including corticosteroids (commonly known as the prednisone-type medications) which can also suppress the immune system, strip the body of bone and muscle, and cause elevations in blood sugar and blood pressure, if left unchecked.

One has to wonder—once most people return to their 20-year-old blueprint, how much less dependence on prescription medication and how much less disability they would have to deal with if they received this approach, rather than the conventional one?

In the next several chapters, I'd like to take some time to educate you about the ***Root Cause Based Medicine using the Youthful Blueprint System***™. First off, it's based on the balancing of hormones. This approach is used to attack weight issues, fatigue issues, and many other basic problems, including depression, anxiety, sleep disruptions and poor coping, through a more structured approach.

Once again, think back to how you felt when you were twenty. Remember how you dealt with weight issues, coping issues and day-to-day stresses when you were in complete hormonal balance? You probably dealt with these issues a lot differently than you do today. In the coming chapters, I look forward to sharing more insight into the Hormone Blueprint System with you, since ***youth is perfect health***.

Dr. Moricz's Six Pillars of Youth

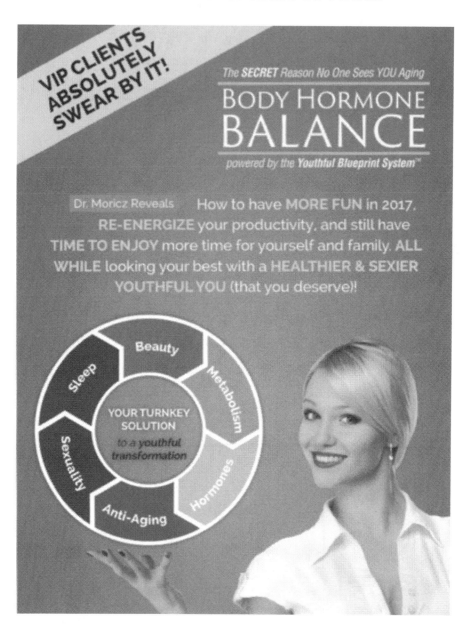

Dr. Moricz's SIX Commandments:

1. Stay on dynamic duo—NAD twice a week shots/lipotropic MIC B12 shots twice a week

2. 3 meals a day, NO snacks

3. No alcohol

4. 12-hour fast (6 PM–6 AM)

5. Proper sleep hygiene

6. Exercise each day (not every other) keep heart rate 130-140 bpm for 30 minutes daily

Chapter 3

Weight Issues

The following are a *collection of interview questions* asked during expert consultations with Dr. Moricz. They have been arranged for ease of reading.

Interviewer: Dr. Moricz, just to remind our audience that two thirds of the adults in the United States are either overweight or obese and, furthermore, there is an unprecedented rise in childhood obesity. Is this really the fault of the American public?

Dr. Moricz: There certainly are cultural and attitude issues toward eating, exercise and weight control. However, from the 1970s and 1980s, the American Diabetes Association took a position on carbohydrates [sugars] that probably contributed more to the rise of diabetes and obesity. More specifically, it was decided prematurely that low-fat diets would be superior to the current dietary recommendations of the time. What this meant was that more than 50 percent of calories would be derived from carbohydrates, or sugar, to create a low-fat diet. It has been shown through weight management studies that low-fat diets have higher failure rates than almost any other type of diet. And for the purposes of our discussion, by encouraging increased carbohydrate consumption, the American Diabetes Association provided the seeds for the rise in overweight and obese adults.

Interviewer: So, are you in favor of restricting carbohydrate sugars?

Dr. Moricz: Well, first it's important to define that there are different types of sugars [carbohydrates] that have different assigned glycemic load and glycemic index values.

Glycemic index and glycemic load reflect how the body's blood sugar will react when different types of these sugars are eaten. So basically, these numbers will give information to people concerned about causing unnecessary sugar elevations in their blood by helping them choose carbohydrates that are less likely to do that. Just as important is looking at other factors that may affect blood sugar levels as well.

First, fiber is extremely important since this might reduce the spike of the sugar after the carbohydrate is ingested. Next, the relative ratio of protein to carbohydrates will often determine how much of an insulin response is necessary to handle the sugar while still achieving appetite suppression. Still, the beneficial use of fats in a diet may actually help reduce the spike in sugar that would be much higher if a person were not to use any fat at all. So, essentially, what is being asked is, *"What is a 'hormonal' approach to weight management?"* This is based not on calorie counting, but on what certain foods do to hormones, such as insulin. There are different ways of thinking about this but consider this—there is a way to eat daytime meals that only minimally elevates necessary insulin levels three times a day—if at all. Put differently, there is a way of structuring an eating plan that may not require the body to elevate insulin markedly through the day and, therefore, avoid the regular effects of insulin on fat storage, while allowing stored sugar molecules to be used for energy burning.

Watch this important video on what I call "Miracle-Gro" for Your Fat Cells:

BodyHormonePalmBeach.com

Interviewer: So, are you focusing on hormones like insulin?

Dr. Moricz: That's right. I realized that whatever system was developed for weight control was really being designed to prevent pre-diabetes and stop worsening of existing diabetes, depending on the person. See, burnout of the pancreas—an organ producing several hormones including insulin—occurs with the consistent carbohydrate challenge, i.e., the typical Standard American Diet (S.A.D.). So, when the American Diabetes Association, medical societies and government agencies encouraged increasing carbohydrates in the 1970s and the 1980s, they were, in fact, promoting what we call *insulin resistance*.

Interviewer: We hear a lot about the connection between diabetes and early aging. Would you comment on this?

Dr. Moricz: There are different ways to explain this but think of the body's poor handling of sugar that results in damage to many cells within the body through a process called *glycation*. Therefore, when a person has syrupy blood, or "too much sugar," sugar is deposited into many cells including nerves and blood vessels, causing damage. One of the ways that the body prematurely ages is by challenging it with too much sugar carbohydrates.

Let's look at it another way. First, too much sugar challenge will overwork the insulin production of the pancreas, which eventually causes burnout of the pancreas.

Secondly, without adequate insulin at the right time [when eating carbohydrates], then sugar levels rollercoaster which forces a person to increase carbohydrate intake because sugar cannot reliably be driven into the body's cells at the right time. So, all of this excessive sugar converts into fat. Insulin has some beneficial role in delivering sugar and amino acids, which are the building blocks of protein, into cells, however, it also promotes fat formation, which is stored as body fat, or as a fatty liver. Ultimately, the continued deposits of sugar into the nerves and blood vessels causes damage which clinically is seen as an increased rate of heart attacks and damage to the kidneys and eyes, among other well-known complications of diabetes. In other words, diabetes accelerates the aging process.

Interviewer: What is the advantage of catching diabetes early?

Dr. Moricz: Look at how many people who are already suffering with diabetes may also have issues with weight control as well. Increased body fat weight is really a symptom of early insulin resistance, or pre-diabetes. That's why attacking weight management from a hormonal approach is the ONLY logical approach to me that is based on solving the original problem.

Interviewer: That's interesting. Dr. Moricz, then do you suspect that is the reason that so many undiagnosed pre-diabetics are showing up at your office with weight control issues?

Dr. Moricz: You nailed it on the head. Aging can be a combination of several processes going wrong. For example, the hormonal changes that a body will undergo as early as the 20's and 30's reflects aging unless it is attacked at the onset.

Interviewer: So, maybe when people say, "You are getting older and your hormones are changing," really what they mean is, "Because your hormones are changing, you are starting to get older"?

Dr. Moricz: Indeed. And I think medicine has really missed the boat on helping people lose weight. And by that, I mean body fat weight.

Interviewer: How so?

Dr. Moricz: For starters, look around at how many commercial programs there are like the ones advertised on TV, print media and the Internet and ask yourself, "Are they really founded on sound principles?"

Interviewer: Tell me more. Does calorie counting really work?

Dr. Moricz: That's an excellent question, and I'm glad that you brought that up. There are really two important definitions that must be covered to understand anything else I am going to say. And these are the two critical definitions: LCD (low-calorie diet) and VLCD (very-low calorie diet).

LCD is an 800-1,200 calorie diet. VLCD is a 400-800 calorie diet. So, a low-calorie diet is often what you see advertised in the media. A very-low calorie diet is a restrictive diet recommended by doctors who practice bariatrics.

These are doctors dedicated to the study of weight management and involved in close supervision of people on these diets. Commercial programs are designed to be low-calorie diets. For purposes of our discussion, restricting calories alone will never increase metabolism and may actually slow metabolism in the long run. A second flaw about counting calories is using weight as the only outcome. All weight tells you is that you are on the Earth and not on the moon. If I wanted to decrease your weight, I would send you to the moon and weigh you. The most important concept that invariably keeps people in the dark is "focusing on weight alone and not body composition."

Interviewer: Interesting, Dr. Moricz. Then how do you account for your success with the *Root Cause Based Medicine using your Youthful*™? How do you teach your clients and get the success that your system is well known for?

Dr. Moricz: You brought up a valid point and I will share the secret that has enabled people to go from measuring a number that is not essentially as important as the next concept that I'm going to discuss, which is body composition. In other words, how do you show people the value of switching from measuring weight to actual body composition so that their success is better monitored, and long-term success can even be achieved?

Well, let me start with a simple example. Take Arnold Schwarzenegger, whom most people know from either the movies or politics, or just from living in the United States. Take someone of his build and frame and have him weighed on a scale at a doctor's office. Well, it's apparent that, based on his height, he actually weighs too much. Next, someone built like him would go to the insurance company to be evaluated by what's called the Body Mass Index, or BMI, which is based on weight, height and surface area. It's obvious that after he is placed on one of these insurance chart tables, which incidentally are often used by many weight management studies and are possibly incorrectly, it is apparent that he is way "off the chart" and will not qualify for health or life insurance. Next, he comes to the ***Root Cause Based Medicine using my Youthful Blueprint System*™**, where we perform a body composition analysis. This measures the actual components that make up weight. In other words, for the purposes of our discussion, the body is broken down into water weight, bone weight, fat weight and lean muscle mass weight. The most important two factors involve fat and muscle content. So, when looking at a person's body comp-osition, the most important thing is to look at these two components.

In the case of someone like Arnold Schwarzenegger, you would find out he is mostly muscle and has very little fat. So, in fact, body composition is more truly reflective of his weight situation and, therefore would be the most accurate way to assess someone at the initiation of a weight management program as they head toward long-term maintenance.

Interviewer: So, do you monitor muscle mass and fat mass, also known as body composition, throughout weight management and hormonal programs?

Dr. Moricz: That's right.

Interviewer: So, what is it that the commercial programs are really afraid of?

Dr. Moricz: They are afraid that most of the initial weight loss is muscle. So, while a person may initially weigh less, they are ultimately sacrificing metabolism because muscle burns calories, even when you sleep. This does not become evident until the weight loss hits a plateau and then patients start to gain weight again, since less muscle means less metabolism and calorie burning. So, unless steps are incorporated to preserve the lean muscle mass through specific approaches, such as nutritional measures and resistance training, the person may be worse off than before initiating the program.

So, in summary, as long as people are kept in the dark and invest in commercial programs that will drop weight without preserving muscle, they will never achieve long-lasting success.

Interviewer: So, I've heard your clients say the *Root Cause Based Medicine using your Youthful Blueprint System*™ not only provides an initial body composition, but continual interval follow-up body composition monitoring that will demonstrate preservation and/or increase in muscle mass while showing continued fat loss.

Dr. Moricz: That is entirely correct.

Interviewer: Comment if you will on the experiences people have shared with you before implementing your Hormone Blueprint System.

Dr. Moricz: One of the large successes of my Hormone Blueprint System is the short amount of time in which it will end incorrect approaches that brought the person to the program in the first place. Put another way, there are four bothersome categories into which people have unwittingly been drawn:

"Group meetings with disenchanted people." Sitting with other people presumes that each individual has a group issue that can be solved with meetings that are not specific to one's metabolism and individualized needs. It is especially discouraging in a society that has the ability to dedicate resources "one-on-one" to achieve acceleration of goals in less time. Because really, that's what we're talking about—time. And in the process of aging, people don't realize that they are losing valuable time for achieving health and avoiding the pains of preventable disease. So, there is quite a bit of wasted time with people sitting in support-group-type formats, when, in fact, the problem is much larger than talking it out, or listening to failed methods of reducing fat by simple changes in diet alone.

"Prepared box meals." There is a disturbing trend in committing people to the repetitive consumption of prepared boxed meals. This is a hyped marketing trend where, in fact, the actual ratio of carbohydrate and protein is not conducive to any success—even short-term success—at all. What it does drive is the need to purchase meals that tout calorie restriction without addressing the hormonal changes that the food composition of the meals encourages. These meals, found both in the supermarket and in advertised programs, need to be better scrutinized. It's unfortunate because by the growing trend of overweight and obese people in the United States, these companies can easily survive, even with a short-term trial of these products, by people suffering with these conditions.

"Calorie counting frenzy." This is an arduous approach, the value of which is even debated among experts. It's very difficult to reproduce even among experts what exact calories, which are actually a unit of heat, for specific foods are among different studied protocols. The other issue is that calories—just like calculating weight mentioned earlier—presumes that the body is absent of hormones, and that the food composition in no way affects hormones. This is, once again, very flawed thinking. It will mislead people into thinking that calorie counting will give them long-term success, when actually the opposite is true. However, it is a big business and probably drives more people to the Hormone Blueprint System based on how discouraged they are with this kind of calorie-counting frenzy.

"Pill clinics." These clinics use appetite-suppressants based on the idea that, if one can restrict appetite and increase metabolism for every client, that this alone will create long-lasting success. Without the structure of an individualized program and careful supervision, however, the use of pills assumes that everyone is similar in their long-term goals and preferences and will respond similarly, both short- and long-term. This approach is equally flawed and will generally be a revolving door of business that usually results in some modest weight control and loss. But as soon as visits are discontinued and prescription weight loss medicines are discontinued, the person is often left helpless. Once again, this fourth category drives a number of clients to the Hormone Blueprint System, which evaluates clients based on their individualized short- and long-term goals, preferences, and realistic monitoring so that they can enter a maintenance phase where they ultimately require less monitoring with a supervising physician.

All in all, these four categories rarely address the metabolism issue and definitely ignore the hormonal one, which requires a deeper understanding and a particular individualization for each person.

Interviewer: I need to ask, what is the secret to the success of the *Root Cause Based Medicine using your Youthful Blueprint System™?*

Dr. Moricz: Well, I do believe there are a number of qualified professional physician experts who are dedicated to weight management. I have simply taken a multi-layered approach that works together for increasing metabolism. Each program is broadly defined as Phase One and Phase Two.

Phase One, regardless of the individual program, is based on fat loss as an outcome. Phase Two is relapse prevention, or maintenance. In other words, once people have completed Phase One, they have achieved their ideal body fat percentage before they can enter Phase Two, which is maintenance of this newly achieved body composition. This is where things get confused in current approaches to weight management. It is only after the target body composition is reached, which is individualized to each client; that a client is allowed to go into the second phase, which is **maintenance**.

I think the reason why I did not involve myself in weight loss earlier in my clinical career is because I had to convince myself that there was a long-term approach to differentiate it from short-term failed approaches. And it was not until I had developed the Hormone Blueprint System that I could address both short- and long-term goals. Ultimately, the client is the outcome, and the body composition speaks for itself. In general, this program works far better for clients who are willing to dedicate themselves to long-lasting goals than for people who are accustomed to short-term success that ultimately leads to long-term failure.

Interviewer: For those people who are not familiar with your background and hormonal expertise, how would you describe how balancing hormones relates to weight control?

Dr. Moricz: I'm glad you asked that question. As you know, youth is perfect health, and when you are able to tune people's hormones back to their 20-year-old blueprint, weight management approaches take on a new level of success. That's why I really believe that it is futile in many cases to even take a multi-layered approach without first considering returning people to their 20-year-old hormonal blueprint. Because think about it again: When you're 20 and you need to lose fat, you certainly can cut back on calories and add some exercise with some incredible results. Taking advantage of that blueprint allows this system to achieve this more quickly, more pleasurably, and with more long-term success. Without understanding the hormonal aspects of weight management, I think a lot is being missed.

www.InvisibleWomanSyndrome.com

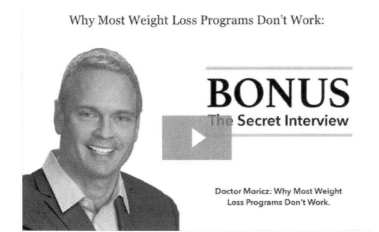

Why Most Weight Loss Programs Don't Work:

Doctor Moricz: Why Most Weight Loss Programs Don't Work.

IMMEDIATE ACTION STEPS

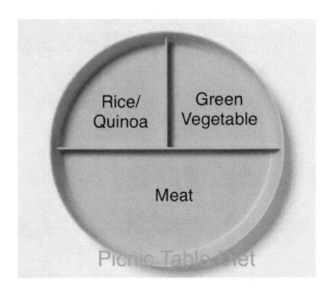

One half of the plate will be meat (or 2 handfuls of meat)/no added gravy or toppings that would deviate from the benefit of unprocessed meat/basically you are using meat that is unprocessed which means you avoid any packaged processed meats, sausages or cold cuts.

One quarter will be green vegetables (not iceberg lettuce or substitutes that are not green vegetables).

One quarter will be either rice or quinoa (not potatoes/also the portion will be a flat quarter of the plate not a heaping scoop of rice like you find in the Mexican or Chinese restaurant).

Dessert which immediately follows consuming everything on your plate will either be a handful of nuts or berries but not both.

You will use the same proportions shown in the pic for both lunch and your evening meal/of course, you can use another choice of meat, different grains and rice or quinoa.

Breakfast could consist of half a plate of eggs or salmon/as long as you have 30g of total quality protein/I discourage use of sausage or inflammatory processed meats/for your carbohydrate 1/4 piece of toast and a handful of berries so that you do not exceed 20g of carbohydrate.

Mistakes that people make is complicating the very simplified Picnic Table Diet/examples include experimenting early on and substituting items that are not listed in the portions above/it may be difficult initially for people to consume a half a plate of meat or equivalent of 2 handfuls of meat which they may need to work up to incrementally/other mistakes include importing ideas where there is elimination of carbohydrates entirely/other mistakes include deleting the dessert which is a handful of nuts or berries or consuming the later as a snack rather than right after the meal/ultimately people who do this will deplete their glycogen stores which they need for energy and will fail.

Other points to remember is that you are eating 3 full meals a day with no snacks/you are not skipping breakfast/and you are leaving 12 hours fasting between your last meal and your morning meal/absolutely no alcohol because that interferes with the breakdown of fat, decreases growth hormone levels, disrupts sleep and is a toxin to the brain as well as a load of sugar which the liver cannot handle and will overstimulate your pancreas.

Vegan/Vegetarian

For those people who are they vegan/vegetarian, there are hormonal and nutritional considerations when designing diet especially the further you are from age 20–10, 20-30 years from 20 years of age. This is often best handled with one-on-one consultation. For those who want to more immediately take advantage of the picnic table diet, they can purchase "Peak Performance Protein" and other products.

Link: Body Symphony Peak Performance Plant Protein | Paleo, Vegan, Gluten-Free - My Body Symphony

https://mybodysymphony.com/product/body-symphony-peak-performance-plant-protein-paleo-vegan-gluten-free/

USE Coupon code: DrMoricz for a discount of 10%

Dr. Moricz's SIX Commandments:

Dr. Moricz's Stay Healthy, Lean and Energized Formula

1. Stay on dynamic duo—NAD twice a week shots/lipotropic MIC B12 shots twice a week

2. 3 meals a day, NO snacks

3. No alcohol

4. 12-hour fast (6 PM–6 AM)

5. Proper sleep hygiene

6. Exercise each day (not every other)/keep heart rate 130-140 bpm for 30 minutes daily

Best of luck using the Picnic Table Diet approach and if you need further involvement i.e. coaching and consulting, please contact us at info@bodyhormonebalance.com

Chapter 4

Sleep and Fatigue

Interviewer: Dr. Moricz, we often hear the terms "tired" and "fatigued." Are they different, or are they the same thing?

Dr. Moricz: Think about this: When you're a small child or a baby and you get tired, you fall asleep without difficulty and get restful sleep that then allows you to be re-energized upon awakening. When adults get fatigued (for several reasons that I will explain later), they have the inability to get true rest and often have many interruptions in their sleep during the night. Therefore, they feel unrefreshed, as if they had never really gotten any rest at all. This is perhaps the most important aspect of understanding the difference between being tired and being fatigued.

Interviewer: Dr. Moricz, we often hear terms related to fatigue, including "fibromyalgia" and "chronic fatigue syndrome." Do these entities really exist?

Dr. Moricz: This is an issue that is still being debated among physicians. I can't tell you how many times physicians will say that there is no such thing as a fatigue-based disorder, such as fibromyalgia or chronic fatigue. I will often ask them, well, do they believe that there is something called migraines, true depression, irritable bowel syndrome and pelvic pain?

They often will reply, "Well, yes, those are well-defined entities, but fibro-myalgia and chronic fatigue don't really have any diagnostic features."

In other words, what they are telling me is that there's really no test because these conditions are diagnosed based on *exclusion*. Well, I can tell you of the above-mentioned problems, they are all diagnosed clinically. And even if one were to try to do diagnostic imaging for migraines and irritable bowel and pelvic pain, it would still be left to clinical criteria and validated pain questionnaires. It is unfortunate that for people who truly suffer from fatigue, be it fibromyalgia or chronic fatigue, that they are still being questioned.

Now, I'm not going to suggest that every person who complains of being fatigued has necessarily met the criteria for these conditions. What I am saying is that, in my work, I have created an approach that will treat the causation of fatigue, so it really shouldn't matter whether it meets the criteria for fibromyalgia or chronic fatigue syndrome, or some other explained reason for documented fatigue.

Interviewer: So, Dr. Moricz, what is the difference then between "chronic fatigue" and "fibromyalgia," and does it really matter?

Dr. Moricz: Well, it does matter from the methodology of medicine categorizing the condition so it can be better studied, and so that studies can further break down subcategories that may not yet have been discovered. In other words, in the process of understanding a disorder, sometimes we figure out there's two or three, or more, variants that need to be analyzed differently and may have different treatments. So, in effect, it really does matter. Practically speaking, there is an overlap of two-thirds of the symptoms between the two entities. And for simplicity's sake, many patients who are labeled with fibromyalgia do have some form of sleep disruption which affects their recovery and energy. Patients with chronic fatigue often have debilitating fatigue that may be related to poor adrenal and immune response.

In other words, they are different and can be categorized differently; however, many times there is quite an overlap of symptoms. So, I often believe that physicians often dismiss things that have not been comfortably diagnosed and where treatment is not necessarily causing immediate recovery.

Interviewer: So why doesn't treatment really work?

Dr. Moricz: Well, let me start by saying that when you break down fatigue disorders, oftentimes symptoms are treated with prescription medications and over-the-counter treatments. In the case of patients with fatigue disorders, oftentimes there is the abundant use of sedatives, sleep aids, antidepressants, stimulants and analgesics under the supervision of a physician. In other cases, over-the-counter approaches, including caffeine-based stimulants and over-the-counter analgesics and antihistamines are used by people looking for a *quick fix.*

Interviewer: Dr. Moricz, help us understand then what is the real basis of these fatigue disorders, and based on that, how does that affect treatment?

Dr. Moricz: That's an excellent question. Let me address a few different issues. Number one: Fatigue-related disorders may include abnormalities in proper sleep function, stress gland hormone production, and related problems, including energy and inflammation. More specifically, these above issues must be evaluated correctly and approached very thoroughly. For instance, sleep is often treated with medications that do not allow for deep sleep.

Number two: Stress gland function is often overlooked with treatments including antidepressants and daytime stimulants. Also, energy function is rarely evaluated correctly with complete neglect of nutritional factors that really do make a big difference. Also, in patients who also have inflammatory changes in the body, including the brain and the gut, without addressing these issues, patients are often in a fog and have difficulty with malabsorption. This further impairs day-to-day functioning and contributes to nutritional deficiencies.

Interviewer: Dr. Moricz, with chronic fatigue syndrome, is there a lot of talk about a possible viral connection?

Dr. Moricz: When evaluating the criteria of chronic fatigue syndrome, it appears there is some compromise in immune system. It is not entirely clear whether patients have sub-clinical infections, such as Lyme Disease that has been incompletely treated, or if there is also an underlying virus.

But the bottom line is that there probably is some compromise in immune system that allows the infections to hover in the body without always producing better recognized infections that doctors are accustomed to treating.

Therefore, analysis of many protocols, such as those involved in attacking bacteria and viruses, will often involve long-term therapy. There are also some integrated approaches that suggest that the body must undergo a detoxification process, which will help the antibiotic and antiviral therapies work better.

So there really is a difference by criteria. However, since many people really don't get treated for these disorders, it's often better to see the whole picture of their fatigue, rather than get caught up in the fact that they may fit one category over the other. As I stated earlier, when you compare fibromyalgia and chronic fatigue patients, two thirds of the symptoms overlap. This makes it sometimes difficult to ignore that they may be variants of a similar disease process.

Interviewer: Dr. Moricz, since you are saying that there isn't a specific test for these illnesses, then what is the recommended approach for evaluating disruption in the patient's functioning?

Dr. Moricz: There are various ways to evaluate fatigue-related disorders. I will mention only a few because the details are beyond the scope of our conversation. Let me start by saying that there is a way to evaluate brain function through neurochemical testing, cellular function by doing intracellular nutrient analysis and hormonal testing to evaluate hormonal disruption. As a follow-up to your question, this then allows for balancing the brain chemicals through the use of nutrient balancing, including the use of intravenous therapy and proper hormonal balancing. The proper use of certain hormones produces an effect called *immunomodulation*, which means regulating the immune system. This is what you do not often hear as an approach. I can assure you that this has been the most valuable multi-layered approach for helping patients with fatigue that I have ever seen.

Interviewer: Having shared what, you have about how fatigue affects people's day-to-day function, why do we commonly hear about weight gain in people suffering these problems?

Dr. Moricz: There are probably three key reasons to explain how sleep disruption affects weight gain. First, in normal patients who sleep well, such as young people, there is a natural rise in growth hormone at night followed by a rise in cortisol levels between 4 and 6 a.m. The growth hormone rise has several benefits, including repair of tissues and breakdown of fat. Cortisol, on the other hand, is a very critical hormone that is responsible for awakening in the 4-6 a.m. period. The problem with patients with sleep disruption is that they have inappropriate cortisol and adrenaline secretion, which disrupts their sleep cycle. Therefore, patients are deprived of the growth hormone benefit for lipolysis, or fat breakdown, along with tissue growth and recovery. Sleep doctors have identified in patients with disruptive sleep a condition of glucose intolerance the next day. In other words, patients' bodies have trouble handling their sugar the next day. This could easily be attributed to the inappropriate secretion of cortisol at night.

Let me also include a word or two about stress gland function. There are several critical hormones that are secreted. The ones of particular importance in this discussion include adrenaline, cortisol and DHEAS. Adrenaline is secreted throughout life and generally until the end of life. Cortisol secretion can be increased, especially under stress. There are conditions under chronic stress where there actually may be a decreased ability for the stress gland to secrete cortisol, even when the stress is resolved. This is called adrenal burnout. DHEAS is an extremely important hormone which is now being linked to immune protection, as well as the ability to deal with physical and emotional stress. It is not uncommon for patients with poor adrenal stress gland function to have a blunted cortisol response and very low DHEAS production. All of this is taking place in an individual who is sleeping poorly and who has poor daytime energy, which often leads to weight gain.

Interviewer: Dr. Moricz, how do patients with fatigue, such as fibromyalgia and chronic fatigue syndrome, present to you when seeking you out for weight control and not necessarily fatigue-related issues?

Dr. Moricz: A very critical approach to patients involves a complete evaluation of their day-to-day functioning. In addition to relevant hormonal and nutritional testing, it is very important to see the common thread between hormonal, nutritional and metabolic issues. Many times, the many people who are seeking me out for correction of their weight loss issues are in fact suffering with energy, sleep and hormonal issues. This is the very point of why I created the *Root Cause Based Medicine using my Blueprint System*: to address the underlying issues for common conditions so that the root of the problem could be better attacked. And in the case of weight, correcting the underlying issues related to fatigue makes reaching a proper body composition far more likely and it will take a lot less time.

Interviewer: Based on the many people whom you see with fatigue, what is the most tragic thing that you often see?

Dr. Moricz: Many times, there are people who will never get the chance to be properly evaluated for their fatigue. I often feel bad because they are not treated well by the medical establishment. In other words, doctors treat symptoms without really understanding that this is a multi-layered issue. And when there is a multi-layered issue, it requires a multi-layered approach. Oftentimes, these patients will suffer not only from some of the problems that we discussed earlier, such as weight, but also develop immobility and ultimately disability. I have seen many patients on pain medications, sedatives and antidepressants, which have further compounded their energy issues and worsened their medical problems.

Interviewer: Dr. Moricz, what is the exact hormonal issue that you have identified and treated in fatigue-related disorders?

Dr. Moricz: Hormones are one of several issues in fatigue-related disorders. I feel that because the hormonal issues have been neglected to such a large degree that it possibly has the most valid justification for being addressed by the right hormonal specialist before other interventions are taken. Specifically, to answer your question, three general areas must be looked at carefully. First, the thyroid; then, the adrenal, or stress glands;

and finally, the growth hormone axis. The details are beyond the scope of our discussion, but they do deserve further analysis. Even when these three hormonal systems are evaluated, oftentimes they are incorrectly interpreted by virtue of a blood test to be "abnormal"—even when the control center in the brain, the hypothalamus, is dysfunctional.

In other words, in medicine, there has been a great deal of attention paid to testing. The context of how the test is being used and whether it truly excludes a problem is far more important. To a clinically experienced hormonal specialist, however, the test is just a starting point. When looking at hypothalamic dysfunction, it often allows the specialist to see how the dysfunction of the control center is causing disruptive release signals to the thyroid, stress glands and growth hormone axis.

So, in summary, there are several hormonal factors for which the correct interpretation is lacking. This subsequently leaves the person thinking that they have been fully evaluated. But I can assure you that, in many cases, they have not. However, when they are properly evaluated and offered treatment possibilities, the results are like night and day.

Interviewer: Dr. Moricz, we often hear about insomnia or sleep-related disturbances. How do you define sleep disturbance so that you can better treat the person?

Dr. Moricz: Based on screening and interview, there are three important aspects of sleep that must be determined. The mistake that I have found over the years is that people are often asked, "How do you sleep?" Because they have become so accustomed to their poor quality of sleep over a long span of years, the answer is often less than satisfactory. What I would suggest is inquiring about sleep initiation, or the ability to get into good sleep, secondly the ability to stay asleep without interruptions or awakenings, and finally how restorative and refreshed the sleep is upon awakening. It is vital that these components be evaluated very carefully. Often the third question about restorative sleep can often clue one into problems not only with sleep, but to patients suffering with undiagnosed pain disorders or nutritional deficiencies.

Interviewer: Then what do you do about the sleep problem once you have identified it?

Dr. Moricz: There is a systematic approach in the *Youthful Blueprint System*™ that I have developed. First of all, the approach has to be individualized to the history and presentation of the person. A detailed review of sleeping habits, medical problems and use of medications is particularly noted. Next, weight issues can often compound sleep issues, such as sleep apnea. This is an important avenue that must be addressed. However, many do not have sleep apnea, but still suffer from very poor sleep. Based on a detailed functional medicine questionnaire review, the issues mentioned above, including initiation, interruption and non-restorative sleep, are diagnosed. Then, based on hormonal, neurochemical and nutritional testing, deficiencies to confirm clinical suspicion is pursued.

If the person has a defined sleep problem based on this detailed review, I use a proven system for building each client an individualized sleep supplement to replenish restful sleep. This has been an extremely successful individualized approach for helping people regain restful sleep.

GEORGE F. MORICZ, M.D.

Interviewer: Dr. Moricz, the more I talk with you, the more I feel that what we are calling medical problems may not really be medical problems at all. Am I taking too much of a leap in saying that?

Dr. Moricz: That's right. Once the neurochemicals of the brain and hormones of the body are balanced correctly, you are no longer in *imbalance*. It would be much better to attack the hormonal imbalance than give a person a premature diagnosis. I cannot tell you how many people I have treated who were once incorrectly labeled as fat, depressed, lazy or poorly disciplined. Unfortunately, they were often flooded with prescription medications by medical practitioners, when in some of these cases it furthered addictions and weight gain problems.

Interviewer: Dr. Moricz, thank you for your eye-opening insight into how you are helping people get restful sleep and youthful energy through your *Root Cause Based Medicine using your Youthful Blueprint System™*.

IMMEDIATE ACTION STEPS

For those of you interested in Dr. Moricz's From Beauty Sleep to Sleeping Beauty Guide – How 6 Years of Poor Sleep Made This Doctor Rethink Everything He Ever Learned in Medical School, please send email to info@bodyhormonebalance.com.

From Beauty Sleep to Sleeping Beauty

How 6 Years of Poor Sleep Made This Doctor Rethink Everything He Ever Learned in Medical School

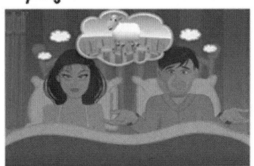

Sleep Right, Every Night and Feel 10 Years Younger Every Day

Discover Your Sleep Blueprint Tonight...

America's Youth Doctor - George F. Moricz, MD

Chapter 5

Why People Aren't Well

In the era of staying well, which translates into peak performance, there is often an over emphasis on losing fat and eating healthy, which by itself is a complement to other vital components that are seldom discussed. In this chapter, you are about to discover why not only is energy, specially produced by little power houses called mitochondria, essential for your body and brain, but combined with blood flow to deliver oxygen, nutrients, and the ability to remove waste, become the focus of peak performance.

In an era where there is focus on fat loss, there is less attention to maintaining muscle - muscle, which you not only had in youth, but gave you all the benefits of youth, especially increasing your metabolism. This goes even so far as helping you take up sugar in the form of glycogen, which is stored in muscle glycogen and liver glycogen, the complex form of sugar. No discussion of metabolism would be complete without discussing uncoupling the storage of calories and the release of heat. Because isn't that really what a calorie is, a unit of heat?

Shortly, you will discover that muscle is not just an accumulation of muscle fibers composed of protein-based molecules. In fact, studies show that loss of muscle, which is called sarcopenia, alters inflammatory biomarkers. What this translates into is that people who have a very inflammatory profile often have a reduction in muscle mass, strength, mobility, and physical performance.

The following interview is performed with Dr. Max MacCloud, who is the founder of My Body Symphony and is known as the Nutrition Ninja Doctor:

Dr. Moricz: Dr. MacCloud, it is a pleasure to be speaking with you, especially since you are the founder of the four M's. Please explain how the four M's become so critical for wellness.

Dr. MacCloud: The four M's, the way I look at them, is what follows after you finish your basics of nutrition and exercise, which are the foundation of your body structure. From there, I look at the four M's as being the key to any chronic disease, especially a chronic condition.

The four M's are the microcirculation or microvascular system, which consists of the capillaries, 99% of your circulatory system. The next M is mitochondria. The mitochondria are powerhouses critical in terms of energy production, no matter what the solid tissue is, which has become more of a focus over the last 10-15 years. This leads us to the next M, which is metabolism, a generally complicated topic in which people get lost.

There are over 3,000 different metabolic enzymes, which when you make it more simple, you start to see how the pieces come together. Since the foundation is energy, what energy pathways should your body be utilizing? There are only three possibilities and two of them are not so good. So, I look at this in terms of insulin and metabolic balance and metabolic activity, building muscle and repair versus building fat.

Additionally, you have your sex hormones, adrenal glands, and thyroid. So, I look at how those fit into metabolism. Next, I look into how you support the metabolism, which utilize hormones and other energetic pieces to balance and strengthen them. However, if the microcirculation is not working right, then you're not getting nutrients to those organs and if the mitochondria aren't working, you don't have enough energy for them to do their job and produce the end products they're required to produce.

And then, lastly, there is muscle. I look at it as a marker for metabolic reserve. It's more than just muscle. I mean, obviously, muscle is critical for adapting to your environment, movement, exercise, which we know determines how you look and feel, but it's also one of the main places that has mitochondria.

Dr. Moricz: So, as you discuss the four M's, the critical question is what happens as you lose muscle, which we call sarcopenia?

Dr. MacCloud: As we lose muscle, which is a cardinal sign of aging, we lose our metabolic reserve.

Look at it this way, and you can prove it to yourself, is as you know, as older folks die from things like flu, well, they've lost their reserve there. Why do anorexics die? Because they burn through their metabolic reserve and then your body breaks down its vital organs. So, probably the biggest aha moment in the 90s with the AIDS epidemic, a lot of progressive docs realized each time one of these people got sick, they lose 10 to 15 pounds of muscle. Well, that means after you finished antibiotics or whatever drugs, they were weaker than before. They have a lower metabolic reserve, and then six, nine months later, they get another infection, which knocks them down another 10 to 15 pounds of muscle. By the fourth or fifth cycle, then they succumb to infection, and they die. So, what they started replacing was growth hormone, testosterone, and using protein supplements, encouraging them to go to the gym and add 10 to 15 pounds of muscle. Sure, you're gonna lose some of that muscle as time moves on, but in the interim period, you have some reserve. So, it became a more survivable condition.

Dr. Moricz: Would you comment on microcirculation?

Dr. MacCloud: So, to focus on repairing and restoring the microvascular system, the microcirculation, we lose somewhere between 50 to 90 percent of our capillaries as we age. The same thing with mitochondria. Over time, people lose anywhere to 40 to 90 percent of mitochondria as they get older, which is a reversible event. And of course, those feed into overall metabolism, keep everything else functioning correctly.

Dr. Moricz: When it comes to the mitochondria, what is so important about that?

Dr. MacCloud: Well, the mitochondria aren't going to work correctly if you don't have enough right nutrients. They're not going to work right if you don't get enough blood supply to the muscles. Every cell has to be within two to three microns from a capillary. Well, if you lose 50% of your capillaries, there's going to be a lot of cells that are not going to be close enough to the capillary to be nourished. So, they start to break down.

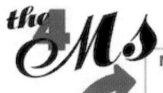

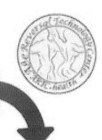

Microcirculation
Makes up 99% of the
Circulatory System!
Feeds Cells & Mitochondria
while Removing Toxins

Muscle
Largest & Most Metabolically
Active System
Primary Metabolic Reserve,
Movement ++

Mitochondria
Site of 95+% of the body's
Energy Production
Energy & Cellular Regulation

Metabolism
Responsible for all functions
of our Physical Bodies
The Sum of all Chemical
Reactions that Allow for Life

Dr. Moricz: So, in summary for our readers, we've discussed the mitochondria of the powerhouses, we've discussed the microcirculation and metabolism, which allows us to burn calories and then muscle as an energy reserve. Now Dr. MacCloud, you've done some special things, not just only to identify these categories but also to support them. Tell me the story again of how you figured out a way to keep people on a diet that's low inflammatory yet supports this system, particularly that of muscle. When people who come to me, they try all kinds of supplements besides food. They try soy, they try whey, which is a milk derivative, and then they try very processed products including pea protein. They go through all these different things, and I don't believe most people are privy to the unique system you developed by figuring out the nutritional benefits of meat and then creating a replacement for it without having to consume meat.

Dr. MacCloud: Sure, as you know protein is the foundation. We're made mostly of protein and needed for repair maintenance and it's also the most expensive of macronutrients to consume because it's metabolically expensive in the digestive process. So amino acids comprise protein - they're the building blocks of our bodies. And there are several sources of course. The politics of people who are pro-meat and animal protein and then plant proteins is obvious in our modern society. People could go either way on that, but from the perspective of what sustainable healthy protein, let me share what I have figured out. We've all heard about whey proteins and rice proteins and egg white proteins and a couple others. Beyond our discussion today is the significance of bioavailability and digestibility. I stumbled across something very interesting with pumpkin seed protein 15 years ago and was comparing them to animal-based products. After six months I got rid of all the other ones because the pumpkin seed protein was much better. It's extremely balanced. It's complete in terms of its profile. It's got healthy fats, and it has all the nutrients you need to be a very complete balanced protein with low allergenicity. So, it's very clean, sustainable protein and then with 11 added nutrients that only occur in red meat, I put them into a pharmaceutical grade pumpkin seed protein product.

> **Dr. Moricz**: To avoid missing anything, you were able to figure out through your historical research about the ancient Greeks and how they were able to perform so well in the Olympics.

Dr. MacCloud: Yes, the ancient Greek Olympians. I looked into the Greek literature and figured out in detail what their diet consisted of, and it's all documented historically. There was a period of 200 years where the top athletes were on an almost exclusive meat diet.

> **Dr. Moricz**: So, what did you do with the pumpkin seed in order to get the equivalency?

Dr. MacCloud: So, I included the 11 nutrients I discussed earlier, basically adding branched chain aminos (leucine, isoleucine, valine) glutamine, alanine, creatine, carnitine, lysine, taurine, protease and vitamin B12. So, basically, I upgraded on a plant-based protein which was missing these important ingredients and developed something sustainable, very clean and good tasting, delivering the same benefits as red meat.

Dr. Moricz: So, for our modern reader of this book, in America they eat what I call ad libitum, a buffet-style ketogenic diet and we know that's not entirely healthy. And then there's other people who do a paleolithic caveman diet. How different is their diet from what you researched and what we're eating in a modern version of either ketogenic or paleo?

Dr. MacCloud: It would be fairly similar, probably closest to the carnivore diet because it really focused on red meat and that led me to look into things that are contained in red meat, not in poultry, not in fish and not in dairy. That's how I came up with the 11 nutrients that only occur in significant amounts in red meat.

Dr. Moricz: So, when I look at your peak performance protein and the nutrients, I will find those in your product?

Dr. MacCloud: That is correct.

Dr. Moricz: And then the reason you were thinking of a substitute because you mentioned inflammation since we're worried about inflammation. You wanted a low inflammatory food, nutritionally that would deliver the same results and bioavailable. Is that correct?

Dr. MacCloud: I wanted something that would deliver the nutrients that a person needs to repair and enhance their performance with as little stress and downside as possible. There are many people who have sensitivities to different foods - a lot of people can't handle whey protein. When it comes to things like grain proteins like rice and pea protein which is very processed. So, there's always issues with those other sources. And with pumpkin seeds, it's what I call the only real food protein powder because it's only two steps. You press the oil from the pumpkin seed and then you grind up the cake that's left. This leaves a product with whole food integrity. Contrast this to pea protein which goes through 14 major processing steps and whey protein which goes through 12 major processing steps. Therefore, they're highly processed foods, totally different than something like for instance a seed like pumpkin which is high in protein and other phytonutrients. What we're doing is knocking down the oil significantly thereby concentrating the protein.

Dr. Moricz: Yes, I've seen people do trial and error in an effort to consume a plant-based protein from hemp, sesame, flaxseed, watermelon, sunflower and yet you don't hear as much about pumpkin seed. So, Dr. MacCloud, as far as the fatty acid composition of pumpkin seeds (Cucurbita), my research shows that it is rich in linoleic acid. The nutritional value of pumpkin and wide range of biologic activity have been known a long time. They are rich in fatty acids, proteins, minerals, and a number of vitamins. The essential polyunsaturated fatty acids perform a particularly important role, especially in cell signaling. Other studies have shown more than 50 macro and micronutrients. Would you comment further from your research and production of this very nutritious product?

Dr. MacCloud: The main oils, as you stated, in pumpkin seed are the omega 6s and some omega 9s and a little bit of the omega 3s. The pumpkin seed protein is still going to retain a small amount of those, but you will draw out some of the fatty acid content when the oil is expressed.

Dr. Moricz: So, you are reducing the fatty acid. In nature, is there a good ratio for us to pursue? Is it ideal to have a 3 to 1 or 4 to 1 or 6 to 1 ratio?

Dr. MacCloud: No, it's not. The only places 3s are in high concentration are in the seed because it comes from plankton. So pumpkin seeds are not a good source, but they have a small amount of omega 3, but mostly omega 6 and omega 9, which in my opinion is fine. But the main thing is that the omega 6s that people are getting in their diet are coming from processed food, so they're altered, they're damaged omega 6s.

Dr. Moricz: Ah, so what you're saying is it's not just looking at the profile of a product, but looking how processed it is.

Dr. MacCloud: Yes.

Dr. Moricz: You're distinguishing between eating red meat omega 6 versus pumpkin seed powder. I guess that is a key take-home point.

Dr. MacCloud: Agree, people can get sick when they're low in omega 6s because they're not triggering prostaglandins, which are cell signaling agents. On the other hand, they can be pro-inflammatory if you receive too much, especially from animal sources. They produce an inflammatory response. Inflammation is the foundation of healing, so someone needs enough, but not too much.

Dr. Moricz: Another point, since we're covering the omega side of things, is you also added amino acids. Was that to give the product the profile of red meat?

Dr. MacCloud: The profile was already very good, but I felt it needed some additional enhancement, so I added branched-chain amino acids to stimulate anabolic activity. Also, I added lysine, carnitine, beta-alanine, and creatine with B12. See, all these 11 components only occur in red meat, all designed to help support the healing and repair process. It's all about building up the tissues.

Dr. Moricz: So, for our readers, there's an anabolic process and there's an anti-catabolic process. What that means with the anabolic process is you're building tissues up, and the anti-catabolic process is the prevention of breakdown, which hormones, especially androgens, have a very important role. This is especially important for people with sarcopenia, low muscle mass, and wasting disease. But here's a critical component, is that you're now saying nutrition that actually has an anabolic effect so you're more likely to stimulate your cells to grow.

Dr. MacCloud: Absolutely. And you need to do it in conjunction with some resistant training, especially as people age, they become more sensitive to mTOR activation of anabolic activity, versus just insulin, because they become more insulin sensitive over time.

Dr. Moricz: Just for clarification to our readers, the mTOR, small m, capital T-O-R, pathway, is a regulator of metabolism physiology, especially supporting the liver, muscle, fat tissue, brain. In other words, genes get activated to create cell protein synthesis.

Dr. Moricz: What Dr. MacCloud was referring to is that as people age, they lose muscle, their insulin does not work as well, and they eventually burn out their insulin. Insulin also has some anabolic effects for supporting muscle, not just stacking on fat in the body. This, along with growth hormone activation of insulin growth factor, is critical because people lose muscle and gain fat. Interestingly, even something as simple as walking after a meal can make you less insulin sensitive, decrease your triglyceride fat levels, and if done long enough, can help build up your muscles.

Dr. Moricz: So, what Dr. MacCloud has offered us is a nutritional way to support muscle growth, which regulates inflammation in the body. Dr. MacCloud, we already have some people who are eating vegan, and they're on board with the idea. What about people who eat meat? They are careful with the Paleolithic diet, and then there's other people who are what I would call a restricted ketogenic diet, which, as you know, we use in cancer. What about the omega 3 component? What should they do if they would like to increase the omega 3 component?

Dr. MacCloud: As a key performance protein, what I do is I add some chia seeds, and that's a good source of omega 3s.

Dr. Moricz: So, the person, without even having to think about it, they're already using your peak performance protein with the pumpkin seed powder, and they can gain an additional source of omega 3s from chia. Is that what you're saying?

Dr. MacCloud: Yes.

Dr. Moricz: So, in summary, this sounds like complete nutrition. This is fascinating. It's low in allergenicity, so people don't realize that they are milk sensitive, and we can talk about how milk is not a natural human source of protein. It's another animal's milk. So, they are using whey protein because of reports of high bioavailability, and then others will use eggs historically because to athletes it's very easy to assimilate egg protein, but here you find that pumpkin seed protein is low in allergenicity, which on food testing egg is not. I see many people are sensitive to one or both components of the egg, the white or the yolk.

Dr. MacCloud: I see people develop sensitivities to foods because they consume too much of it and they don't digest it efficiently. Not too many people consume too many pumpkin seeds because it's considered a superfood for years, and by concentrating the protein portion of it but still maintaining it as a whole food, I do not come across anyone that was sensitive or allergic to pumpkin seeds. Alternatively, other foods have been concentrated or highly processed and they develop sensitivities, and I think that's the issue, especially with dairy.

Dr. Moricz: Dr. MacCloud, so many patients might say, well, why don't I just chew on a bunch of pumpkin seeds, but I understand that besides being organically sourced, that the outer shell of the seed could be a source in other pumpkin seeds of pesticides. What are your thoughts on that?

Dr. MacCloud: Well, you are right. We only use organic and certified seeds, but the thing when chewing pumpkin seeds, you're going to tear your gums after a while, and they get stuck between your teeth. It's a limitation of that type of consumption consistently, but if someone has a tolerance to it and can eat enough of them, I say go for it.

Dr. Moricz: In summary, Dr. MacCloud has shared his system on the four Ms: microcirculation, mitochondria, metabolism, and muscle. He's also provided us with not only the background but also the solution for people who want to stay well and not get sick.

IMMEDIATE ACTION STEPS

By now you realize the importance of muscle mass. There is a difference between body mass index BMI which looks at more at volume than it looks at the individual components of muscle, bone, water and fat.

BF% body fat percentage is important but more important is skeletal muscle mass (or lean body mass)

Your immediate action plan is to undergo body composition analysis. The gold standard is DEXA scan.

However, an impedance-based body composition analysis such as that shown below can also be used with great reproducibility as long as your hydration is similar between each session.

There is no need to check a body composition more than once a month.

There is almost no need to be checking the scale more than weekly which may only show weight and does not differentiate between muscle, bone, water and fat composition.

Let's take a look at two charts below to give you a visual.

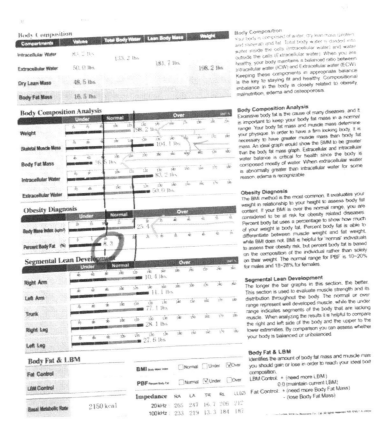

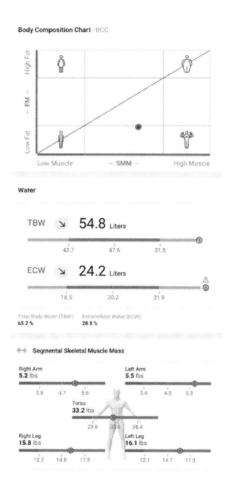

Referring to the body composition examples shown above, you will see:

- Weight

- Skeletal Muscle Mass

- Body Fat Mass

- And Water Composition (both intracellular and extracellular)

- Body Mass Index

- Percentage Body Fat

The goal is to have a body fat percentage between 10 - 15% in men and 20-25% in women. The goal with skeletal muscle mass is that it be above average, and the body fat be below average as you can see in the chart.

Bonus:

For those who want to more immediately introduce their body to the benefits of organic pumpkin seed powder discussed in this chapter, they can purchase "Peak Performance Protein" and other products.

Link: Body Symphony Peak Performance Plant Protein | Paleo, Vegan, Gluten-Free - My Body Symphony

https://mybodysymphony.com/product/body-symphony-peak-performance-plant-protein-paleo-vegan-gluten-free/

USE Coupon code: DrMoricz for a discount of 10%

Chapter 6

Why People Stay Sick

Everywhere you go, people are talking about cleansing and detoxification. With good intentions of eliminating toxic exposures, introducing nourishing foods, and a healthy lifestyle, people use the word detoxification in a very well-intended way. People are aware that the body has its own mechanisms for detoxification. From the skin, liver, kidneys, digestive system, and respiratory systems, the body uses these organs to break down and eliminate toxins from the body. With the challenge of a massive amount of toxic exposures and pollution in the environment, it makes sense to enhance the natural detoxification of our organs.

Obviously, everything from heavy metals, mold-related mycotoxins, chemicals, herbicides, pesticides, and air pollution contribute to the toxic overload in our lives. People will often use methods including infrared saunas, exercise, supplementation, including antioxidants and detoxifiers, IV therapy, and numerous supplements. What may come as a surprise is that, like most things, if not done in the correct order, it may not have the intended benefit. The most frustrating cases I see on a daily basis involve clients who experience side effects from detoxifying in the wrong order. Many are not even aware of how people can recirculate toxins that were intended to be excreted through the bowel, but instead recirculate through what's called the enterohepatic recirculation through the liver, which puts a great deal of strain on the body.

Furthermore, there are biofilms which act as a layer used by organisms which prevent most of the usual practices of detoxification from becoming effective. This barrier is seldom discussed and rarely addressed. Even worse are people who use toxic binders without having prepped the systems that we are about to discuss in this chapter.

In an era of why people question why they can't get better, the obvious question is why they aren't initially well. In an effort to reverse biological aging, there is a consumer market chasing wrinkles, sunspots, gray hairs, the classical signs of aging, by trying to address exposures such as ultraviolet radiation, chronic stress, and lack of sleep. More importantly, the issues of toxin exposure and toxic burden often need to be directly addressed. There is something called the exposome, which is the environment of toxins to which people are exposed throughout their lifetime. This is known to accelerate biological aging by disrupting the normal cell processes that are intended to maintain our health. There is another term called Gerontogens, which include air pollution, smoking, and heavy metals.

Our understanding of proper detoxification may be the most essential concept for our health. You will discover how proper detoxification needs to be done before other anti-aging regenerative therapies are instituted. Conceptually, when your body is detoxing correctly, systems such as the liver, kidney, digestive, and skin are used to break down and eliminate toxins from the body. Unfortunately, the overload of toxins flooding into our environment combined with our modern-day lifestyles have compromised these detoxification pathways, which means our bodies are unable to process and excrete toxins effectively. What happens often is consumers will try things online and in health food stores which do not consider a problem called the enterohepatic recirculation. What this means is that toxins don't end up being 'bound' for excretion through the bowels, but instead go through multiple cycles of processing through the liver, reabsorbed through the intestines, and recirculated by the liver.

Compounding this is biofilms. This can be thought of as a protective coating used by organisms to prevent detection by your immune system. This is especially problematic when these harmful organisms reside in your gut lining and use heavy metals and other sugar substances to create a physical barrier. Testing will often not be able to detect organisms because of these biofilms.

In summary, environmental toxins can be categorized as heavy metals, mycotoxins, chemicals, herbicides, and pesticides, as well as air pollution. This is why we must be careful about the air we breathe, the fluids we consume, the foods we eat, and the products used at home and on your body. What we will discover is there is a more ideal order in which detoxification can be supported, which if not done this way, results in frustration and delayed improvement in your health.

The following interview is performed with Dr. Brian Yusem, who is the founder of HEALUS Health:

> **Dr. Moricz**: It is with great pleasure that I interview Dr. Brian Yusem, the founder of HEALUS Health. In particular, we will be exploring why people are so sick, especially as it relates to detoxification. As many people have read, the liver, skin, digestive system detoxifies at one point in life better than at another point in life. Based on all the systems that you have created, what is the biggest problem you see when people come to see you for detoxification?

Dr. Brian Yusem: Well, most people don't have a clear idea of what detoxification, or the ramification of detoxification really is. There are problems with methylation factors and gut function for releasing toxins. Specifically, getting them prepared for release from the body. For instance, in heart disease and plaque aggregation, we find that females do very efficiently with plaque removal and males do not because they don't have the proper methylation factors to unleash toxins to get rid of them from the body.

Dr. Moricz: What Dr. Yusem is referring to is the transfer of carbon molecules, particularly as a signal for detoxification of the liver. Methylation can also affect the way that hormones, brain chemicals, and the DNA signal as well. Additionally, in America, the number one killer is heart disease, and the number two killer is cancer. So, if someone came to a naturopathic doctor like you for education on how to rid the body of toxins, they may really be thinking, I don't want to get heart disease and develop cancer. So, they might be asking, can I take a substance and make it bioactivated, which makes it more soluble - make it a little more dissolved in water? Then number two, if I can neutralize it, hook it up to something and conjugate it, that would be really cool in the liver. And then thirdly, I'd like to transport it out of the body – elimination. When they come to you, Dr. Yusem, what kind of detoxification are you recommending and in what order?

Dr. Brian Yusem: Well, I precisely do what you're saying because they need to understand what detoxification is and what it takes to rid the body of toxins. Our immune system is efficient the way it stands from the moment you are born, and you need to allow the immune system to do its job that it was designed to do like it was years ago. People may not know this, but compared to ancient times, we now have 22,000 toxic chemicals in the environment and 12,000 in our food. People are eating fake foods, breathing fake air, and everything is destroyed.

Dr. Moricz: So, you said something interesting, something historical. I always believe and I describe that youth is perfect health, but maybe in our modern civilization, this has changed. When do you believe, like you said, in ancient times, there was a shift in our ability to handle environmental loads?

Dr. Brian Yusem: This happened when our society became more industrialized with chemicals. Back in ancient times, they had exposure to minerals, things they would etch things out of, and they drink out of copper and drink out of certain metals that were quite toxic. In Roman times, particularly in Sardinia, Italy, before they had earthquakes, they uncovered all the toxic metals they were drinking from urns which they were manufacturing. This seemed to start the wave of toxification and toxin overload. People were not detoxifying and unable to live in health for 30, 40 years as a population.

Dr. Moricz: So, returning to what you were saying, people have a kidney system, they have a liver system, they have a digestive system and have a respiratory system, which in Chinese medicine over 4,500 years, was the basic efficient system needed for detoxification. In the life cycle of a human, using the naturopathic approach, by what age are you finding that people are starting to gunk up their body and become less efficient?

Dr. Brian Yusem: We're seeing this very early. We're seeing it pass from blood values in our air samples. We're seeing from male and female counterparts that are giving birth to toxic children. And, depending on the toxic loads given through birth, it can be variable levels of toxicity. Well, the toxicity of water was done years ago and showed 50 times the level of these endocrine disrupting chemicals, particularly plastics. Just as general knowledge, people hear about plastics abbreviated PP, PVC, HDPE, polystyrene, PET or PETE, LDPE and ABS. Environmental chemical analysis shows how this can disrupt normal hormonal activity and plastics that are in our food now, like Baskin-Robbins ice cream, are being consumed without people even thinking about it.

Dr. Moricz: As a historical perspective, we have an all-time low in males of male hormone levels, low sperm counts, and in females, overstimulation of sexual development, including the breast, bleeding issues, and triggering of autoimmune conditions, where the body attacks itself. Dr. Yusem, you mentioned Baskin-Robbins ice cream. For anyone who goes to a diner or restaurant, they're also being bombarded with Morton salt, which has plastic-like compounds in it as well.

Dr. Brian Yusem: Absolutely.

Dr. Moricz: Just as an additional insight for our readers, what Dr. Yusem is describing is if you believe your body's working great, you're going to realize it's not because if you don't optimize your detoxification, you'll have more inflammation, immune disruption, and you will disrupt the way that you make hormones and neurochemicals. So, a number of people will come to us, and they'll say, "I've done a detox." What kind of simple detoxes are you seeing that are really incomplete?

Dr. Brian Yusem: Well, they're selling an empty bag of hearsay because they're not getting detoxed very well whatsoever. I have rarely seen people eating properly. And then there's natural substances like cilantro and different natural herbs that may work, and they may also be using residuals from volcanic ash and fulvic acids that you can liquefy or eat some in purified form that will chelate or remove chemicals from the body that are riding hard on your immune system.

Dr. Moricz: So, a lot of people say, I'm doing a detox of sort. They do some kind of diet. They do some kind of prep like you said. And then other people are getting caught up with these binders. As an example, things are like a gourmet meal. They have to be done in a certain order, period. As you were developing your HEALUS system, you have an algorithm which you're going to share. And what I have found is that in speaking with you and other experts that people jump in the middle of a process, and they don't do things in the right order. By way of example, they go in for chelation to bind up heavy metals. And then once in a while, a practitioner will say, wait a second, but you have a high fungal load, and then they're low in glutathione, and they're high in mercury and cadmium. Discuss for us the order of how you figured out how to detoxify the body.

Dr. Brian Yusem: Yes, that's a good question. First of all, the biggest elimination system next to your skin is your digestive system, so that you need to make sure that your digestive system is working properly to rid yourself of toxic compounds. And secondarily, we need to go after yeast and fungus and things that cause yeast and fungus to grow or expand or aggregate in your system where they're starting to cause a problem.

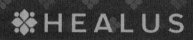

8 CLEANSING PHASES

1. DIGESTIVE CLEANSE

Your gut houses 85% of your immune system. Commonly referred to as "the second brain", your gut is arguably the most important organ system in the body. Our Digestive Cleanse will heal your stomach lining, increase healthy bacteria growth, and balance to the rest of your body.

2. CANDIDA CLEANSE

Candida is "too much of a good thing" in action. It commonly presents as brain fog, a weakened immune system, or symptoms of leaky gut. This happens when a particular kind of yeast becomes too prominent in the body. Our powerful, herb based Candida Cleanse is designed to eliminate bad bacteria, soothe inflammation, and improve your mood.

3. PARASITES CLEANSE

Studies show that over 80% of all Americans have parasites. Common types of parasites include, ringworms, tapeworms, hookworms, etc. If affected, you may experience skin issues such as rosacea or cystic acne. Other signs include inconsistent bowel movements, poor sleep quality, and fatigue. Our Parasite Cleanse will not only kill the parasites, but the eggs and larva as well.

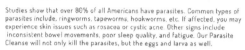

4. LIVER CLEANSE

The liver is the largest internal and most metabolically complex organ in our bodies. It performs over 500 different functions including fighting off infection, neutralizing toxins, manufacturing proteins and hormones, controlling blood sugar and stabilizing healthy body weight. Our Liver Cleanse will reset hormone levels and revamp thyroid function.

5. HEAVY METAL CLEANSE

Heavy metals can find their way into your body by way of drinking water and things like, pesticides, alloys, and steel. Heavy metal toxicity commonly presents as brain fog, confusion, and fatigue. More serious conditions such as Alzheimer's can develop if toxicity goes untreated. Our Heavy Metal Cleanse eliminates metals, and alleviates anxiety and depression.

6. HORMONE BALANCE

Your hormones affect every part of the body, from your energy to your confidence, emotions, and sex drive. Our Hormone Protocol will aid the healing of your adrenals, thyroid, and hormonal function, while adding a LOT of pep to your step.

7. PHYSICAL FITNESS

Diet and proper nutrition are a vital part of a healthy lifestyle. Equally important to your ultimate health and mind-body wellness is your physical fitness. It's not just about looking good, it's about your body moving well, feeling good, and being strong.

8. EMOTIONAL FITNESS

Studies have shown that the heart is 60 times more powerful than the mind energetically. This means that getting your emotions centered is transformational in itself. Creating a consistently healthy emotional state elevates your health both biologically and the way you feel about life.

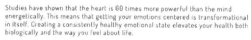

WWW.HEALUSHEALTH.COM

Dr. Moricz: So just to recap, step number one is to make sure the digestive system is working properly. So, this would mean improving what we call phase one and two of the liver and then also help in elimination. Is that correct?

Dr. Brian Yusem: Well, it's digestive elimination because we do liver detoxification a little bit later in the system.

Dr. Moricz: Oh, that makes sense. So, the first is to improve bowel flow in the colon.

Dr. Brian Yusem: No, not colonic. It needs to be, but it needs to be out of the small lumen of the small intestine and the large intestine (the colon).

Dr. Moricz: So, everything after the stomach. So, in other words, small bowel to large bowel first, which is very important, and then number two, you said once that's moving, you'd like to hit the fungus and then parasites. Is that correct?

Dr. Brian Yusem: Well, we do the fungus because the fungus is really an issue that people don't recognize, and it's the metal composition that causes the chemical toxicity where the metal holds the fungus in a state of compromise. Basically, you never get rid of fungus unless you get rid of chemicals.

Dr. Moricz: So, what you're saying is number two, you attack the fungus. Is that right?

Dr. Brian Yusem: Right, you never get rid of it, but you can lower the loads.

Dr. Moricz: Because we have colonization, a healthy person with a balanced immune system, they also have parasites. What I mean is they have bugs in there, including lots of bacteria. What you're talking about is over colonization of fungus. Is that correct?

Dr. Brian Yusem: Yes, and you'll never get rid of that with one approach.

Dr. Moricz: So, what you're doing is decreasing the load in step number two, and then parasites?

Dr. Brian Yusem: Yes, number three is parasites.

Dr. Moricz: So, you're deciding that the fungus would be more important to take care of first because you want some parasites to live in the gut.

Dr. Brian Yusem: Yes, it's a natural function of the living organism to have a healthy balance of parasites and bacteria.

Dr. Moricz: As an example, there was a lot of water damage in the last couple years in parts of Florida, which saw a peak of prescriptions of itraconazole, which for many years was used for toenail fungus, and that's a pretty nasty antifungal, and as you may realize, Dr. Yusem, is that people have been taking this six months or a year or forever. I mean, they've been cycling this forever, and then on top of it, they were taking ivermectin, a deworming medicine since COVID. What are your thoughts on all this as it affects the microbiome, the environment of the gut?

Dr. Brian Yusem: I totally agree with you because they'll never get rid of it, and I've seen, I've had people on it since Second World War, and they have toenail fungus, and they never got rid of it, even if they treated it at the site. You need the, the magic word here is momentum, and you get ahead of it like a wave, and you want to surf on the front of the wave and take care of the toxic detoxification principle and keep it coming out of your body gradually with a proper momentum over time.

Dr. Moricz: So, what you said is important - momentum. You're doing phase one for a small, large bowel, which makes sense for transit, so do you continue the process while you're hitting the fungus, transitioning to parasites, and so on, or do you overlap them?

Dr. Brian Yusem: Yes, you keep the momentum going because you'll never forget what it feels like to rid the body of toxins and see them come out of your body, and what they look like if you can see them, period. There are millions of parasites, and they look like pieces of rice with a little head, a black head on them.

Dr. Moricz: Now what I found in my own practice is that Candida can be very persistent in the gut, and you made an important point. You're just trying to decrease the load. It's very difficult in the gut. Vaginally, you can get rid of it. Orally, you might get on top of it, and the skin, it's a little easier to get rid of it, but what I've also seen, heard, and recommended is a use of hydrocolonotherapy. Do you ever introduce that at any point in the colon for people heavily loaded with Candida?

Dr. Brian Yusem: At the tail end, if people want to get rid of it and they can do it hydrocolonically, yes, that's an option. They can use MSM to choke it out, choke out the parasites and get rid of them.

Dr. Moricz: Oh, for the parasites - I was referring to fungus, so MSM, the methylated compound, methyl sulfonyl methionine. Now, we're continuing the process, the GI cleanse, correct?

Dr. Brian Yusem: Right, you don't stop there, you're going to go into the liver and start cleaning out the toxins you've collected over these phases. In the liver, because the liver is responsible for 500 different detoxifications. It's time to clean up the liver now. Usually, people can feel differently as soon as they start detoxifying liver. You'll never forget what that feels like, it's a total release. You feel lighter and your body's lighter and more efficient and think clearer. You don't have brain fogs and things like that.

Dr. Moricz: That makes complete sense. I know in the Oriental system they look at the liver, gallbladder, bowel system first, then they do kidney, bladder, and then they do toxins, pathogens, which you know I attribute a lot to respiratory issues, but going back to your point, in your expertise you've developed expertise in another area. We were both independently developing a glutathione and butyrate suppository before we met. How do you use this in the liver detox? Because people can get sick during a liver detox, and I have even used IV nutritional Myers cocktails during detoxification.

Dr. Brian Yusem: Yes, you can do that with suppositories, you can use glutathione suppositories.

Dr. Moricz: That is interesting because I have used IV glutathione with nutritional support, alpha lipoic phosphatidylcholine, and you developed suppository support that you can add during the liver gallbladder detox.

Dr. Brian Yusem: The advantage is it goes in like an IV, which you can do daily, maybe over the course of a month, and it's $150 for a liver clearance IV, where for suppository it's a much smaller investment.

Dr. Moricz: So, what we're talking about is using glutathione, and for the reader there's two processes a little beyond the scope of our chapter, where the first makes it water-soluble or bioactivates it, and in the second step it neutralizes it, it conjugates it. Stated differently, you have to hook it up to something to get it out of the body, and what Dr. Brian Yusem has described is a very elegant, easy way you can do at home by using a glutathione suppository to support the process. Alternatively, I have seen people who either flushed out too much or get overwhelmed without glutathione support and get very sick. Have you seen this as well?

Dr. Brian Yusem: Yes, I have, and you bring up a great example when you want to chelate metals, you've got to detox the bladder and kidney. So, this is step number five, the kidney bladder step, for which I've developed special detoxification herbs that have been used for thousands of years that effectively clear out the bladder and gallbladder, which people are forgetting that you need your gallbladder. You don't want to get rid of your gallbladder that's responsible for assimilating all the fat in your body, otherwise you won't be able to digest fats.

Dr. Moricz: And then are you continuing your special suppositories during that process?

Dr. Brian Yusem: You can do them simultaneously - people use glutathione throughout that, and there are other dietary considerations to help the body detox from having issues with the gallbladder.

Dr. Moricz: So, in Ayurvedic medicine, what Dr. Yusem is describing is that there are certain ways to eat and the order in which you eat is important for detoxification. In the American burger fries' diet, people say, I'm doing intermittent fasting, they eat crap all week and basically this doesn't make any sense to the body. You can't starve yourself twice a week, hit yourself with alcohol, which is very disruptive to the body. That is not detoxification. That's how you toxify yourself, and it loads the liver with fructose, which makes it very difficult to detoxify. So, the diet he outlines in his systems is what you eat the way you eat. See, like I said earlier, this is like preparing a gourmet meal for a restaurant. You do it in a certain way. You don't just make it up. And I think that's what we see happen. People say, I'll do a detox over the weekend as if it's a casual thing. It's a commitment.

Dr. Brian Yusem: It's a way of life.

Dr. Moricz: So far, we've gone through the steps to get you back to a new normal, and then there's maintenance. But if we allow the body to toxify to the point that it needs help, you have to un-toxify it. So, what we've identified is all the steps leading up to the kidney bladder. Dr. Yusem, tell us more.

Dr. Brian Yusem: Well, the metals are a piece of the puzzle, and you want to stay on a chemical detox. I do hair sample analysis and hair mineral kits, and then you find out where you start, and then you do chemical detoxification. And then I use a light detoxifier and a heavy-duty detoxifier.

Dr. Moricz: So just so we don't get lost, in your algorithm is number six metal detox, is that correct?

Dr. Brian Yusem: No, you're right. There's metal detox, and that's where I use fulvic acid, and magnesium EDTA, which is less caustic than sodium EDTA.

Dr. Moricz: That's right. The big danger he's talking about is the type of EDTA that you use, period. You use a magnesium EDTA.

Dr. Brian Yusem: That is correct.

Dr. Moricz: So, what Dr. Yusem is describing is that some people have access to an IV clinic, and they can get an EDTA binder, a chelator to remove them, but they have to remember that removing other metals that are needed in the body can be disruptive. People ask, why are heavy metals problematic anyway? Because they take the place of usual minerals that help your enzymes move. Enzymes are sort of the protein we don't talk about. They're the ones that make all the reactions in the body happen. So, we're talking about metals like mercury, cadmium, arsenic, lead. Do you have other ones that you commonly see in your testing?

Dr. Brian Yusem: Well, those are the basic top ones. And for that, I use these volcanic derivative binders.

Dr. Moricz: Now, so in your system, we are at the point of detoxifying after metals. So, after the chelation part of detoxification, do you try to tune up hormones?

Dr. Brian Yusem: There's an interesting thing that happened, is that because the immune system is the most efficient in your body, once you get rid of the residual toxins in the body you're speaking about, at some point, your body will perform hormonally and functionally much better. You don't have to concentrate on symptoms. You just go and do the system. And then at some point, many things will drop off.

Dr. Moricz: What Dr. Yusem is describing is when you reduce cytokines or inflammation in the body, then hormones work better. As an extreme example, for people who can afford to just get trillions of stem cells, and their hormones work better. I've seen this discussed at conferences. The reason is because the inflammation went down, the releasing hormones and stimulating chemicals from the brain, they work better. So, it's sort of like if you tune up your hormones, inflammation goes down. And then if you reduce the inflammatory cytokines, then the side benefit of reducing inflammation is your hormonal systems work better. As a side point, earlier we discussed the use of glutathione. It is an immune regulator. So, when people go into what's called TH2, which I call more of an allergic immune response, when they have COVID, Lyme or autoimmune diseases, what happens is that with the use of glutathione, it tilts you back to TH1, which is where you want to be balanced. So, it's an important immune agent. So, if somebody takes advantage of this, they could be modulating their immune system. Notice I said not boosting it. Boosting could create an autoimmune effect, which is often not a good idea.

Dr. Brian Yusem: Yes, because you're cleaning up the adrenals at the same time, this is the fundamental starting point to your hormonal pathways combined with proper eating style and not fasting. I'm not a believer in fasting myself.

> **Dr. Moricz**: I usually have people do a 12-hour fast, a lighter dinner and a bit heavier lunch so that the natural melatonin in their gut can release, you detoxify, you can activate all the anti-aging pathways and there are a half a dozen of them. So basically, what we're trying to do is boost our ability to recover and get rid of bad cells. The term used is autophagy.

Dr. Moricz: In summary, this has been a fascinating interview with Dr. Yusem in this chapter on how someone can properly approach detoxification with the simple certainty that by working with the right practitioner, they could be getting the results they need. Alternatively, it's hit and miss, trial and error with you getting sicker and not being able to detoxify your body.

IMMEDIATE ACTION STEPS

Bonus:

For those of you who would like to reap the benefits of the HEALUS 8 PHASE Detox reviewed in this Chapter.

Save 15% when you use Discount Code MoriczMD at:

https://healushealth.com/products/gut-health-bundle-cocoa

Chapter 7

Why People Get Dementia

Let's start with - what is dementia? Dementia is defined as an acquired disorder that typically involves decline in cognition. We can think about cognition as the process of acquiring knowledge and understanding things in life through thought, experience, and the senses. Scientifically, cognition falls into the category of learning and memory, language, executive function, complex attention, perceptual motor, and social cognition. In the psychiatric and neurologic evaluation of dementia, the requirement is 'only' that one of these areas have a substantial decline.

The form of dementia that we most commonly hear about in older adults is Alzheimer's disease, which accounts for 60-80% of cases. Something discussed outside of the doctor's office is mild cognitive impairment, which is a gray area between normal cognition and dementia, where there are defined impairments, but not an overall decline of function. Current science, believes the neuropathological process of dementia begins 15 to 30 years before obvious clinical symptoms, which may be a window of opportunity of detection and prevention. As we will learn later in this chapter, although dementia was once considered incurable, some forms of dementia may be reversible.

As we will also discover, previous approaches to dementia have been largely unsuccessful because of delay in diagnosis and failure to identify the underlying disturbance. A one-approach system usually doesn't work because the final diagnosis is a common pathway of multiple disturbances in the body. Around the world, it is thought that dementia cases will triple over the next 30 years, the largest of which is Alzheimer's disease. Currently, 6 million patients are affected, and it will cost over a trillion dollars by the year 2050 for supportive care of patients suffering with Alzheimer's. This is not to mention the devastation it causes not only for the patient, but family members as well.

It is my honor to interview Dr. Joshua Helman, an expert in dementia and reversal of this horrific diagnosis. Dr. Helman heads up a dementia reversal center in the Palm Beach County of Florida and has extensive background in research and clinical intervention for patients suffering from dementia:

> **Dr. Moricz:** When patients present, they're certainly not admitting that they have all the changes in the areas of cognitive function from learning, memory, language, and complex task performance. With what complaints do patients usually present?

Dr. Helman: Normally when I see patients, they don't say, 'Dr. Josh, I have dementia', they say, 'I feel like I have brain fog', 'I have low energy, I can't do the things I used to be able to do.'

Dr. Moricz: So, when they come with these complaints of brain fog, share with us how many different types of doctor expert practitioners do they see before they end up with an expert like you?

Dr. Helman: 10, 20, 30, up to 50, including people with the biggest names out there, including Cleveland Clinic, Harvard, Yale, Mayo Clinic. Yes, they have been going to big places, including the head of a chair department, and they feel as if no one can help them.

Dr. Moricz: Okay, then people will say, especially family members, you know, it seems like this is the normal part of aging, because traditional medicine says mild cognitive impairment is considered part of normal aging, where in fact, substantial memory loss is not. Others may be asking; do they have depression? Is this related to another condition? What comments do you have about that?

Dr. Helman: Every case is a little bit different, but in most cases, I've evaluated is multifactorial. In other words, it's not just one or two things. It's normally 10 up to 30 causes, including toxins, infections, inflammation, including genetics, sometimes it's head trauma and vascular problems, period. But every case is a little different, and I see whole families with the same symptoms, and then it may be that you're dealing with predisposing genetics plus toxins, infections, living in similar environments.

Dr. Moricz: So, Dr. Helman, what you're saying is that depending on how they present, when they present, is we may be oversimplifying by labeling it with a name - kind of putting it in one basket, whereas you're saying there are a lot of different underlying reasons that weave into each other and produce what people are simply bumper-stickering as dementia. Is that a way that we might be thinking about it?

Dr. Helman: Yes, that's exactly right. Added to this is another frustration because they've already been to dozens of doctors and expert places where they're not getting help. In fact, sometimes they're just being labeled by doctors 'you have a psychiatric problem, the simple test we did on you was normal and obviously you're not functioning well, and therefore they may be malingering or presenting as depression or some other psychiatric condition because the test that was done looked normal.' And obviously they're not functioning well, so we'll call it a psychiatric condition.

Dr. Moricz: So, you're saying that in traditional medicine we work in silos and specialties, and we may be forcing a diagnosis or excluding something a little too early or maybe a little too simply. Is that possible?

Dr. Helman: That's exactly right, and I feel the whole system is set up for simplicity. And sometimes simple is perfect if you have a simple problem like a laceration of your skin, that needs to be sutured. If you have an isolated problem like that, let's say you have a large exposure to mercury, a one-time exposure to mercury, and you fix it by doing chelation (binding up the metals) then their brain returns to normal functioning. But often it's not just one problem, it's more complicated. By the time I see people, the simple cases have already been filtered out.

Dr. Moricz: So, there can be an accumulation of exposures, toxicities, and processes in the body, which is why traditional medicine is not adequately able to address it?

Dr. Helman: Yes, that's entirely possible, and that's what I find happening in most cases.

Dr. Moricz: Okay, so people throw out numbers. Okay, we hear the word dementia being defined as some decline in cognitive functioning, depending on what that might be. We hear about memory lapse or the loss of memory as one of the earlier signs. How should we be thinking about these problems?

Dr. Helman: There are really four types of memory problems. First, there's the four-second memory that's focused on the frontal lobe, the lateral aspects of the lateral lobe, and we can see that on the PET scan of the brain, where if it's working or not, but then there's also the conversion of the four-second memory to the four-hour or the four-day memory. So, someone could have a very good four-second memory, which you can appreciate when you have a conversation with them, they feel like they're completely with you until you ask them what they had for dinner last night and they have no clue.

Dr. Moricz: Very interesting. As you know, as a specialist in emergency medicine, people present and just want to have one kind of test that would identify the entire issue. What do you think the future of neuroimaging is, or is it being used correctly, period? Is it used early enough, or have we dismissed it because we're not offering the higher-level SPECT, PET scans, or a focused MRI imaging?

Dr. Helman: Yes, the functional MRIs and PET scans with neuroquantic imaging are definitely extremely helpful when measuring the function of your brain, but unfortunately, they are viewed as experimental. So normally the only imaging studies that my patients have before I see them are structural scans, specifically an MRI or CAT scan of the brain, which you know is helpful to find a structural problem like a bleed in the brain or a tumor. That's extremely useful, but in most cases, the scans are normal.

Dr. Moricz: I can appreciate that. Backtracking a little bit, I see people in their middle to early years, early 60s, when their speed and memory, which you know I define as youth, is compromised. One of the areas that I find disrupted is sleep. People lack youthfully restorative sleep. How much do you think that sleep disruption contributes to aging of the brain, and if we were looking at the brain as a communication of nerve cells and connections, how disruptive or contributive is this to dementia?

Dr. Helman: Yes, from the artificial intelligence machine learning data, it turns out that analyzing patients with Alzheimer's or other dementia categories, it turns out that poor sleep and specifically deep sleep disruption problems are the biggest risk factor for developing Alzheimer's and other dementia.

Dr. Moricz: Dr. Helman, you mentioned AI, which everybody hears about artificial intelligence, and we're curious what is the latest and greatest on how we're going to use AI to help us with diagnosing, treating, and maybe even stratifying dementia. As you know, what is the best approach to learn about how to use data so that we don't have to rely on trial and error or our own experiences for sharing information?

Dr. Helman: Yes, AI is a tool, but like a lot of other tools, it's only as good as the information that has been inputted. One of the challenges in clinical medicine I've seen firsthand is that the way data is collected is not even accurate, which is unfortunate, but basically you need to look at the primary data, you need to look at previous treatments and previous diagnostic studies to tease out what's actually going on.

Dr. Moricz: Your criticism, so I understand correctly, is that you mentioned the applicability of AI, which is limited critically by the data that's inputted into the AI. Is that correct?

Dr. Helman: Yes, that's what I'm saying. Imagine seeing a patient that has already been treated by 12 different large medical institutions. First, getting all the records from these 12 places can be challenging because they're working on completely different systems. Once you obtain these records, sometimes the information in the records is not even correct.

Dr. Moricz: So, as you mentioned earlier, AI could definitely be used, but let's say we could work with someone like Elon Musk, okay? And we had all the resources in the world, what do you think would happen? How are we going to use AI in a world of dementia? How do you think we could use AI better?

Dr. Helman: Yes, so what I'm concerned about doing, number one, is making sure the clinical information about the patients in the data set is complete and accurate, so that's number one.

Number two is using imaging technologies to measure function of the brain immediately after each type of treatment. For example, one way to measure how well your brain is functioning is to perform a mini mental status exam. Another is a quantitative EEG and measure your brain function.

And then the other factor includes new medical modalities that can help us over time, depending on whether the treatments we are doing are helping or not helping the outcome.

Dr. Moricz: So, if I'm understanding correctly, you would be a proponent of standardization of certain measurements through the life cycle of not only the patient's illness, but actually the interventions themselves.

Dr. Helman: That's true, and the analogy I would use is that if you have some unsettling heart problems, you can measure their EKG and know, not 100%, but with pretty good accuracy and sensitivity, whether they're currently having problems with their heart or not.

Dr. Moricz: That's an excellent point. So even if the diagnosis was made earlier and if we agree with the statistics, currently it is stated that somewhere between 60 to 80% of what we call dementia is Alzheimer's disease. Is that over-represented or is that about accurate?

Dr. Helman: Actually, if you look at the people over the age of 65, closer to 80% of adults will have Alzheimer's disease.

Dr. Moricz: Alzheimer's disease. And for the reader, that means we have some either biopsy-proven or chemical or deposition of plaque, am I correct on that?

Dr. Helman: Yes, fatty plaque or biofilm. But what's exciting is that there are newer tests, whether imaging or blood, where you don't necessarily have to do a brain biopsy to get a diagnosis. But I think the other important thing to be up front with people is even though right now we have a number of different neurological degeneration modalities with completely different names, whether multiple sclerosis, ALS or Parkinson's or Alzheimer's, when you explore that list, then I would advocate looking for root causes of the problem.

Dr. Moricz: So, what I have read and seen, Dr. Helman, is that Alzheimer's can be broadly characterized as five different insults - brain inflammation (either due to chronic or infection), and others including toxicity (due to exposure of heavy metals, man-made or naturally occurring toxins), deficiencies in factors such as hormones, nutrients, and vascular, and traumatic injuries. Is that correct?

Dr. Helman: It turns out that if you look at the root causes of a number of these above noted diagnoses, they turn out to be identical. They are the same types of toxins or infections. It just happens for whatever reason that men are more likely to get degenerative disease called ALS and women are more likely to get disease of MS or Alzheimer's. So, what I'm saying is that it's great that neurologists have very specific clinical criteria, but I think we're missing the boat because the root causes for many of these clinically disparate, very different diseases are actually the same.

Dr. Moricz: Basically, the background environment, the exposures, will drive the process to a point in the decision tree and then at one critical point what you're trying to uncover with either AI or good data collection is that there's differentiation. Stated differently, it takes a different path.

Dr. Helman: Yeah, that's part of it. What I'm saying is that 10, 20, 30 years from now, when we reflect on our current paradigm approaches, we're going to laugh. To me, it's comparable to the way physicians practiced 100 years ago where the response for every disease was to collect blood, you know, get leeches out, and drain people's blood.

Dr. Moricz: So a lot of what you're saying, too, is that if these earlier exposures may ultimately be common to all of these disease processes, then if we had an earlier way to detect using AI and if this was done more perfectly, then we would introduce this intervention earlier in life so that we may be able to attack some of these exposures and risks with the possibility of deterring the disease process. Am I being too optimistic?

Dr. Helman: No, you're exactly on the right track, but what we have found so far from AI is that often in the case of Alzheimer's, the symptoms, you won't get symptoms until 10 years before the clinical presentation and the symptoms will start slowly.

However, you can actually go back and look at different causes that started 30 years previously, which of course you weren't really aware of until maybe 20 years later.

So, what I'm trying to say is that just because someone right now is functioning normally, they may have things lurking under the visible level which the body specifically has high levels of redundancy and it's only 95% of the backup, it's only when 95% of the backup systems are destroyed that people say, 'oh it's like my brain is not working today'.

Dr. Moricz: So, in summary here, a lot of the exposures and pre-symptoms, pre-overt symptoms may be common for other disease processes as well, and the same exposures are also causing other illnesses. What besides diabetes would be another pathway that we should look at for attacking this issue before symptoms present?

Dr. Helman: So, one of the common root causes besides Alzheimer's and other dementias, diabetes and other conditions like cancer, vascular problems, is actually inflammation. Inflammation and an overactive immune system are the common root causes for all these problems.

Dr. Moricz: For the reader, we often think about inflammation as something being in the immediate phase and then there's chronic inflammation. Certainly, you need acute inflammation (the short phase) to fight off injury, infection, or to fight off exposure to toxic substances. People may think of that as pain, redness, swelling, and heat in the body. Chronic inflammation, on the other hand, is really what we're talking about.

The other factor mentioned by Dr. Helman is an overactive immune system, which means that we have an early invader system and then we have a more long-term invader system. We have memory of antibodies in our system and then we have something called T-cells, which is made in the thymus gland, which basically allows us to not succumb to illness.

We often hear about an overactive immune system, especially if the body attacks itself or if somebody has constant sensitivities to the environment. So, do diabetes, sugar, insulin issues promote the progression of these illnesses?

Dr. Helman: That's very true, but my point is it may just contribute to one dementia in 20 or 50 different dementias.

Dr. Moricz: With regards to treatments, particularly in the database of Alzheimer's drug discovery, we hear about the latest, which I will have you comment on. Most people have heard about the current treatments including cholinesterase inhibitors, NMDA receptors, blocking these and other monoclonal antibodies, MAOs, and vitamin E. Update us about the most current approaches.

Dr. Helman: So far, we haven't talked about galactin-3. This is a pro-inflammatory molecule for which we now have FDA approval for compassionate use as a drug to promote Alzheimer's reversal, basically by getting to the root cause inflammation and blocking it.

Dr. Moricz: So, for the reader, galactin-3 belongs to a family of what we call lectins, which are sugar-binding proteins. This is very involved in cell signaling, which we've often heard about in inflammatory conditions and as a biomarker for cardiovascular disease. In wound healing, it activates immune cells. When it gets dysregulated, especially in a variety of cancers, it becomes a target for cancer immunotherapy.

What I think you're about to explain for the reader is that it is elevated in neurodegenerative diseases, especially the more severe the disease is. Part of the issue is penetrating the blood brain barrier, which we understand is the area that you have to get past in order to be effective. Studies have shown elevation of the galactin-3 levels in Alzheimer's, Parkinson's, ALS, stroke, and even delirium, which is a short-term disturbance, sometimes confused with dementia.

Tell us about your focus on inflammation. Is this the reason they are using this type of drug?

Dr. Helman: Yes. Although every case is a little bit different, and there isn't one magic bullet that's going to fix everything, we still have to go to the root cause first.

Dr. Moricz: As you go to the root cause with your unique background and expertise in dementia, would you also offer this therapy which works on the galactin-3? How would you describe this to our reader so they could understand it better?

Dr. Helman: If you could visualize the immune system and how we need an immune system, a functioning immune system, to help us heal wounds, to keep out bacteria, but specifically by blocking inflammation triggered by galactin-3, we are basically able to tone things down and put our body back into homeostasis (balance), and in this case, improve brain function.

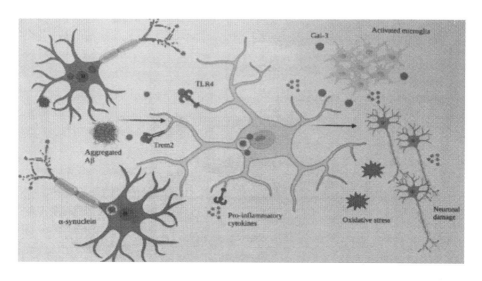

Illustration of cellular dysfunction in aging and neurodegenerative disease

Dr. Moricz: In summary, Dr. Helman has presented a fascinating preview of what is likely to happen in the future in the reversal of dementia. Especially with his description of inflammation that may be presenting 30 years in advance while traditional medicine is waiting for the check engine light, which sends us scrambling to attack the diagnosis. By reducing the inflammatory response and using the benefit of data, especially through AI correctly, this would be extraordinary for improving the lives of so many people.

IMMEDIATE ACTION STEPS

If you are suffering from brain fog, signs of dementia or are at high risk for dementia based on medical history including family history, then I recommend testing for mycotoxins and heavy metals & toxins.

It cannot be emphasized enough the importance of quality sleep for which you may find more information in chapter 4 of this book.

Also be sure to follow Dr. Moricz's SIX Commandments on daily basis:

1. Stay on dynamic duo—NAD twice a week shots/lipotropic MIC B12 shots twice a week
2. 3 meals a day, NO snacks
3. No alcohol
4. 12-hour fast (6 PM–6 AM)
5. Proper sleep hygiene
6. Exercise each day (not every other)/keep heart rate 130-140 bpm for 30 minutes daily.

Chapter 8

Why People Get Cancer

Cancer is known as a large group of diseases that can start in any organ or tissue in the body when abnormal cells grow uncontrollably beyond their usual boundaries to invade other parts of the body and spread to other organs. We often think about cancer as being caused by changes to DNA, particularly damage to the DNA.

Beyond the scope of this chapter is proper diagnosis for a selected cancer from a certain organ and therapeutic interventions, both traditional and complementary. Most people know that there are risk factors for certain cancers, including tobacco, alcohol, lack of exercise, unhealthy food, extra body fat, family history, and environmental exposures. In developing countries, infection plays a significant role for cancer deaths, specifically human papillomavirus, helicobacter pylori, and hepatitis B and C viruses account for over 90% of infection related cancers. In developed countries, the top five cancers include lung, colorectum, breast, stomach, and prostate cancer.

It is my honor to interview Dr. Thomas Bige,
Founder of the Reboot Program in Ocala, Florida:

Dr. Moricz: With me today is Dr. Thomas Bige, founder of the Reboot Program in Ocala. We will look at less heard of, yet very significant perspectives on why is it that people get cancer and don't recover as they could.

So, people will often hear about traditional reasons that people get cancer, whether it's a light switch, a genetic predisposition, an environmental trigger, and so forth. But tell us what you think, especially with your varied backgrounds in naturopathic medicine, traditional medicine, and stem cell therapy. What is the perfect storm for someone to develop cancer?

Dr. Bige: The number one is lack of emotional fitness. Like the capacity of a computer, the mind must protect against invaders such as viruses and fungus. We do have proof of most cancer and that it's driven by fungal infection.

Dr. Moricz: You said fungal infection, is that right?

Dr. Bige: Yes, it's infection. It's the biggest pandemic in the world.

Dr. Moricz: Initially you said emotional fitness. For people reading this chapter, is that something that's programmed by four years of age? Is it the way they cope, their habits?

Dr. Bige: Capacity. The capacity to deal with environmental negative effects.

Dr. Moricz: So, adaptability, the ability to adapt to the environment. Is that another way to look at it?

Dr. Bige: Adaptability, but mainly in a Western world, people's emotional adaptability is restricted to the environment. They don't have to fight on a daily basis, which means the sensors, the level of excitement from a negative stimuli is increased.

Dr. Moricz: So, in a world where people are not overexposed to social media, television, computers, and they live more by survival, war, tragedy, poverty, limitation of resources, does that train their brain differently?

Dr. Bige: Absolutely. The value of distress is paramount. In the Western world, people get stressed out because they get 'too hot' coffee at Starbucks.

Dr. Moricz: So, our expectations are important.

Dr. Bige: Expectations, yes. We have to pay for the comfort that's created, and the payment is that our system is not reactive first against all invading intruders as much as if you were walking barefoot on the street.

Dr. Moricz: So, the fungal part, when people think of fungus, they think of infection rather than colonization. And as you know, for thousands of years, we have parasites, we have fungus, we have them in different parts of our body. What particularly can you explain about fungal overgrowth, candida? Explain a little bit about that.

Dr. Bige: Yes, Candida is thought of as nasty stuff. Candida is just a Latin word for yeast and that is good yeast and bad yeast. If the yeast gets trapped in the digestive system more than 24 hours, it runs out of oxygen and if there's mold around it, we learn how to utilize nitrogen instead of oxygen. Utilizing nitrogen becomes the problem because it's used instead of oxygen.

Dr. Moricz: In a previous discussion, we talked about first lines of defense against all organic pathogens that come in food and the way to attack organic pathogens, whether it be using ozone-infused olive oil with food, coconut oil. We are trying to combat anaerobic pathogens (those that survive without oxygen and oxidize viruses). The most effective way to reduce yeast mold colonies in the colon is colonic irrigation with ozone-oxygen infused water. Because the yeast mold overgrowth in the colon causes anaerobic fermentation of carbohydrates which produces alcohol and methane gas, the alcohol attacks the liver and causes dehydration in the kidneys. The gases reabsorb into the blood and end up in the lungs. The lungs are used to utilizing oxygen from air to deactivate the methane that causes inflammation which significantly reduces oxygen availability to the blood. Besides avoiding antibiotics, excessive sugar, and environmental disruptors, what could we be doing to decrease our candida load in our gut?

Dr. Bige: To use up the consumption of the carbohydrate sugars you eat in your diet. Since the preferential form of energy in the brain is sugar in the natural form, the body protects it. If you reduce sugar to zero in your diet, your mental function declines without this energy resource. Not that the sugar is the problem. The problem is not utilizing sugar as energy and the liver is forced to turn it into fat cells.

Dr. Moricz: As our clients may know, if you take sugar and you hook it up to fatty acids, you have what's a triglyceride (fats). Is that what you're talking about?

Dr. Bige: Yes, that's correct. A simple way to think about it is if you exercise enough, you could even consume donuts. If you don't, you can't have any excessive sugar at all.

Dr. Moricz: What you're saying is that if we increase our metabolic demands, we basically dissociate the release of calories versus the storage of calories.

Dr. Bige: That's correct. And when you look at the small intestine unloading semi-digested carbohydrates, mainly man-made carbohydrates to the large intestine where the yeast colonizes and pumps out multiplication of yeast cells into the bloodstream. This can travel for three months before it returns to the large intestine. In the meantime, during its travels, the yeast thrives on the sugar, creating blood sugar fluctuations which can be the basis for many other problems, including the feeding of cancer cells or formation of cancer cells because the brain keeps regulating the pancreatic beta cell production of insulin when the yeast fungi suck on blood sugar.

Dr. Moricz: For our readers, people read about glucose and fructose, and then of course, if they eat more natural sources like fruit, which has higher fiber, but the question is, it's not the glucose, it's the fructose in the artificial foods that the bigger issue. Am I correct on that?

Dr. Bige: The fructose, again, you need to look at it in two ways. Fructose is more dangerous in a way because there are monosaccharides and disaccharides (simple and more complex sugars) and the effect on the liver is far more extensive than having something fattier like donuts. Donuts have a combination of both lipid fats as well as sugars.

Dr. Moricz: Donuts because of the fat or because of the sugar?

Dr Bige: Because the sugar intake of the flour, the flour, which after the fructose is unused - very high in carbohydrates - which attacks the liver as it gets processed through the liver if you don't turn it into fat, which then causes damage to the liver. It's a heat thermal effect of the sugar in the liver which then forces the liver to produce cholesterol, LDLs. That's what the big deal is, not the cholesterol. The cholesterol can be cleaned out with quercetin, in things like raw onions, for example.

Dr. Moricz: So just to clarify, quercetin. Which you noted is contained in raw onions, for instance.

Dr. Bige: That's why simple people eat onions and apples after fatty food.

Dr. Moricz: What if they cook with onions?

Dr. Bige: The cooking makes it different. Cooked onions facilitate melting stored fat.

Dr. Moricz: So, there is a thermic effect.

Dr. Bige: Yes, a thermic effect. The enzyme in the raw onion has a scraping of cholesterol deposit in the arteries and veins.

Dr. Moricz: Here are two different uses of the same natural substance.

Dr. Bige: Absolutely.

Dr. Moricz: Earlier you mentioned the emotional component. We also talked about the fungal load and the big theme, of course, of calculating your metabolic thermic needs as opposed to how much you're intaking carbohydrates.

Dr. Bige: It's very simple. After eating two slices of bread, you're supposed to walk two kilometers or say one and a half miles.

Dr. Moricz: I see.

Dr. Bige: That's the bottom line. Then it's absolutely no problem to have two slices of bread.

Dr. Moricz: Now this exercise needs to be done right afterwards, correct?

Dr. Bige: As soon as possible.

Dr. Moricz: Because of the insulin effect. Because triglycerides are lowered and insulin sensitization. People are thinking, I'm worried about cancer. So, I work on the emotional component, which we can talk about later. We reduce the sugar load and then the fungal component. Give us a third big one that's leading to cancer.

Dr. Bige: It's the fear from cancer.

Dr. Moricz: Okay, so the fear, does this not go along with number one?

Dr. Bige: The problem is lack of emotional fitness, which causes the cancer sickness. And then the medical establishment telling them they have cancer, and the fear sets in. That's why it doesn't fit quite in the emotional fitness group because it happens afterwards. It's a paralyzer.

Dr. Moricz: When people come to see me in functional integrative medicine, they're loaded with metals, mycotoxins, and then they don't get enough oxygen and nutrients and antioxidants. Would you consider that a background effect that leads to more cancer?

Dr. Bige: Absolutely with the nutritional deficiencies. That's why I do hair follicular scanning, which is a specialized hair analysis. For the person who's new to this, it's based on what's called homeostasis (balance) and then epigenetics (the way the environment affects the DNA). The information is based on plucking hair follicle bulbs from the rear of the skull. This ultimately results in a personalized nutrition report on 12 key indicators, plus analysis of the gut, immune, circulatory system, as well as resistance and environmental indicators.

Dr. Moricz: Please tell us more.

Dr. Bige: Once the sample is taken from the skull, from the C1 vertebra, which is unique to a special hair follicle which regrows every three months. Then it is decoded using hair follicle bulb information sent through a Tesla coil via satellite to Germany. There they use a supercomputer to analyze the code, which yields a 30-page packet of information helping us tune up the patient's nutritional state, antioxidants, minerals, and even level of emotional pressure.

Dr. Moricz: For the reader who has never heard about this information, information is coded in vibration just like the sound of my voice, whether you use wireless or use a remote control to open your garage door. Ultimately, the information is decoded looking at these vibrational frequencies and then use it to correlate it with physical nutrition deficiencies and excesses.

Dr. Bige: Yes, that's correct. You can even determine the amount of sleep the person has through that time.

Dr. Moricz: That is interesting. How would they accumulate all this data and reverse-engineer it to a gold standard? How did they do that?

Dr. Bige: They decode the information through a Tesla coil. The analog software works on particular areas using AI technology. This can be done in any office anywhere and send the samples in specialized mail. With special equipment, the coding and sending of information to Germany is done in 30 minutes with the results available to the doctor and patient.

Dr. Moricz: So once again, a theme that we have been discussing in this book is that number one, at an earlier point in life, before somebody develops metabolic illness and cancer, we could be intervening. My professor in college in the 90s, Dr. Thomas Seyfried wrote a book Cancer is a Metabolic Disease. While he was not using these technologies, he described how disrupting the mitochondria with excesses of sugar and creating fat in the body was sending signals to the DNA, damaging signals to the DNA. Would you comment on that as being consistent with our discussion?

Dr. Bige: That is part of the answer. Of course, the weakened cellular system is more susceptible of getting invaded by the invaders, the causative infectors. There's a disruption in the magnetic field. In other words, if I take a tribe member from Kenya or Lake Victoria and place that person in New York for a month, that person can develop cancer.

Dr. Moricz: Are you talking about electromagnetic fields?

Dr. Bige: For example, it's just part of the dirt, part of the pollution, because everything that nature provides to those tribal members is protection, even if they get a snake bite.

Dr. Moricz: So, if someone stays in their untouched environment, their non-contaminated environment, it's protected, but this changes once they come to the westernized world.

Dr. Bige: That's because there's enormous pollution in the United States.

Dr. Moricz: When you say pollution, people think of air. People think about the air, but you're also talking about chemicals, insecticides, heavy metals. Am I right? Am I missing something?

Dr. Bige: Food, drink, air, and emotional pollution. The cumulative effect can cause cancer because there's nothing natural about it.

Dr. Moricz: So, when we often think of primitive cultures, and I'm not degrading them, what I'm saying is that we think they're surviving and we're thriving. Conversely, in a modern society, it may be in reverse, that they are thriving and we're surviving because of the environment. Is that correct?

Dr. Bige: Yes, that's correct.

Dr. Moricz: So, the person who comes here and listens to this and they're concerned about their emotional component, their adaptability, they're concerned about fungal overload, they hear what you're saying about the environment. When they visit someone like you, at a minimum you would test a hair analysis and so forth. We may also be thinking of preventable things for the person who doesn't have cancer, who may not have obesity, who's not taking medications or toxifying themselves on purpose, but lives in a modern society, sits in front of a computer eight hours a day, and goes home and does a little more of the same. What components do you think they could easily fix?

Dr. Bige: Number one, it's adequate sleep that's allowing the immune system and nervous system to repair itself from all the damages incurred during the day. Not allowing it to accumulate. If the person has deep restorative sleep, the amount is adequate. Because of what we call the body clock, developed by the Chinese. Every two hours, different organs get serviced. Some of them need conscious, and some of them need subconscious service, and some need a combination of the two.

Dr. Moricz: In concluding, what Dr. Bige has described as the Chinese medicine's 24-hour body clock, divided into 12 2-hour intervals of vital force moving through the system. This is based on the concept of cyclical ebb and flow of energy through the body. The 2-hour intervals Dr. Bige discussed helps restore the body. This system can be traced back to as early as the year 960.

CHINESE BODY CLOCK

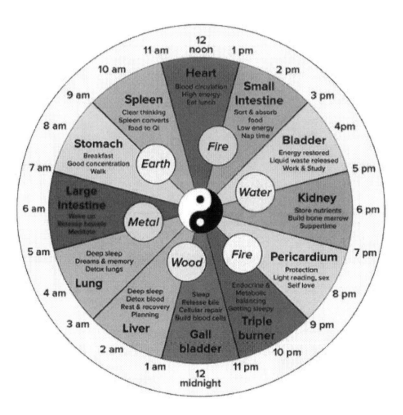

https://www.healthline.com/health/chinese-body-clock

Conclusion

Thank you for joining me on this very intriguing journey of why people do not get better. As promised, we explored why people decline, biologically age, get sick, and show up to the doctor's office. Not only have we covered why youth is perfect health, the reason that you had youth in the first place, but also the changes that the mind and body undergo when it loses youth 10, 20, 30 years later.

You also discovered why traditional approaches are failing, especially waiting for the signs of inflammation to accumulate in the body. You also enjoyed fascinating interviews on metabolism, nutrition, detoxification, dementia, and cancer, as well as the role of AI in the future of medicine.

Many of you are asking yourselves, what if I want more? For those of you interested in exploring more in video format, please go to www.bodyhormone.com. For others of you who enjoy podcasts, feel free to go to **www.GeorgeMoricz.com**.

And still others of you may have questions, which if time allows, could be sent to **info@bodyhormonebalance.com**. Whatever you do, please share the contents of this book with family, friends, and people with whom you would like to enjoy a much bigger life.

With all the health, wealth, and success that life has to offer you.

George F. Moricz, M.D.

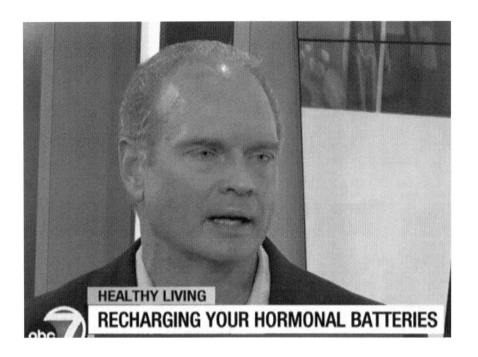

IMMEDIATE ACTION STEPS

If you are at risk for cancer, diagnosed with cancer, or recovering from cancer, I recommend testing for mycotoxins and heavy metals & toxins.

It cannot be emphasized enough the importance of quality sleep for which you may find more information in chapter 4 of this book and the role of proper diet and weight control to keep the body free of cancer cell stimulation further discussed in chapter 3 of this book.

Also be sure to follow Dr. Moricz's SIX Commandments on daily basis:

1. Stay on dynamic duo—NAD twice a week shots/lipotropic MIC B12 shots twice a week

2. 3 meals a day, NO snacks

3. No alcohol

4. 12-hour fast (6 PM–6 AM)

5. Proper sleep hygiene

Exercise each day (not every other). Keep heart rate 130-140 bpm for 30 minutes daily

About The Author

George F. Moricz, MD

Concierge Regenerative Medicine Doctor

Founder of the Youthful Blueprint System™

Dr. Moricz earned his medical degree at the University of Massachusetts Medical School. After a rewarding career in pelvic surgery and infertility, he expanded his offerings to his clients, including medical bariatrics, anti-aging medicine, and energetic medicine. His creative work including innovations in skin beauty systems, natural sleep systems, and nano energetic formulas.

Attracting clients from around the country and overseas. Dr. Moricz proudly offers individualized and customized blueprint systems to help his patients heal and live a fuller life. As an international best-selling author, Dr. Moricz released *Body Hormone Balance Revolution* and the *Hot and Sexy Hormone Solution*.

For those interested in having Dr. Moricz speak or provide training to other practitioners, please send email to info@bodyhormonebalance.com.

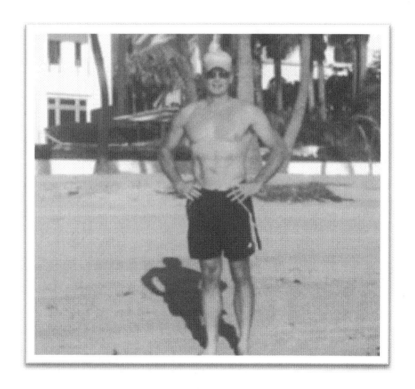

Made in the USA
Columbia, SC
01 April 2025

56022539R00076